Red Light Therapy:

Unlock the Hidden Power of RedLight for Pain Relief, Energy & Anti-Aging

Peakstate Protocols

FREE BONUS FROM PEAKSTATE PROTOCOLS

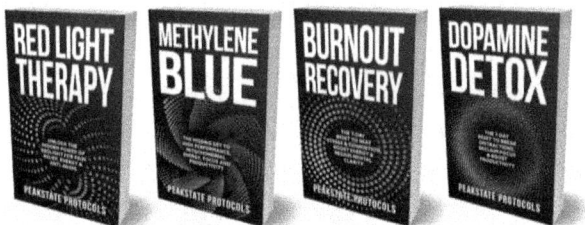

TABLE OF CONTENTS

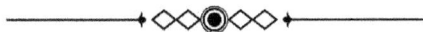

Introduction

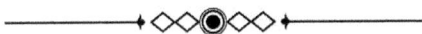

——◆◇◇◉◇◇◆——

I remember the first time I tried red light therapy.

I was standing in my bathroom, feeling slightly ridiculous as I held what looked like a science fiction prop up to my face. The gentle warmth spread across my skin, bathing everything in a deep crimson glow. Part of me wondered if I had fallen for some elaborate wellness scam—another shiny gadget destined for the graveyard of abandoned health fads in my closet.

But I was desperate. Months of mysterious inflammation, energy crashes at 2 p.m., and skin that seemed determined to age faster than I was living had left me willing to try almost anything. So there I stood, bathed in red light, wondering, "Is this actually doing anything?"

That was three years ago.

What happened next wasn't a miracle—let's get that out of the way right now. I'm allergic to miracle claims and overnight transformations, and you probably are too. But what did happen was a gradual, persistent improvement that I couldn't ignore. First, my sleep improved. Then, I noticed how quickly I recovered from workouts. Eventually, even that stubborn patch of psoriasis that had resisted every cream dermatologists had prescribed began to fade.

I'm going to guess you picked up this book for one of two reasons: Either you're curious about whether this red light therapy actually works, or you already have a device gathering dust somewhere because you weren't quite sure how to use it effectively. Either way, you're in the right place.

Here's the problem with most health innovations: The gap between the science and practical application is often Grand Canyon-sized. On one side, you have researchers publishing exciting papers about cellular mechanisms and statistical improvements. On the other, you have regular people just trying to figure out what to do on a Tuesday evening to feel better. The bridge between these worlds is often shaky at best.

This is especially true with red light therapy. The research is genuinely fascinating—we're talking about using specific wavelengths of light to enhance the way your cells function at a fundamental level. But when it comes to actually implementing it in your life, most resources either drown you in scientific jargon or provide instructions so vague that they might as well tell you to "just shine it and hope for the best."

I spent nearly two years down the research rabbit hole (my partners and friends can attest to how I became that person who couldn't stop talking about "photobiomodulation" at dinner parties). I tested different devices, protocols, and timing strategies. I tracked results obsessively. Most importantly, I connected with hundreds of other red light users—from elite athletes to grandmothers with arthritis—to understand what actually works in real life, not just in laboratory settings.

What I discovered was both simpler and more nuanced than I expected. The benefits of red light therapy are real and backed by significant research. However, the difference between people who see transformative results and those who do not often comes down to the consistent application of specific protocols—knowing exactly what to do, for how long, and in what order.

That is why this book is not structured like a traditional health book. You will not need to wade through 100 pages of theory before getting to the actionable content. Instead, I will provide you with a 30-day framework that anyone can follow, regardless of their starting point or specific health goals.

Think of this as both a map and a flashlight for your red light journey. The map will show you exactly where to go, while the flashlight will illuminate why certain paths matter more than others.

A quick note on the whole "wellness industrial complex" concept: I understand. We live in a time when it seems like every day brings a new must-have health gadget or supplement promising to revolutionize your life. It is exhausting, expensive, and often disappointing. I am not here to tell you that red light therapy is the answer to all your problems or that you need to spend thousands on equipment. In fact, I will show you options that fit various budgets, including some surprisingly effective DIY approaches.

What I am promising is intellectual honesty. When the research is strong, I'll tell you. When it's preliminary or contradictory, I'll tell you that too. Red light therapy isn't magic—it's a tool. And like any tool, its effectiveness depends on how and when you use it.

So whether you're dealing with chronic pain that has limited your life, skin issues that affect your confidence, energy problems that impact your work, or simply a curiosity about optimizing your health, I've designed this book to meet you where you are.

Over the next 30 days, we're going to transform red light therapy from a confusing, high-tech concept into a simple, effective part of your routine. And unlike so many health interventions that feel like punishment (I'm looking at you, ice baths), this one actually feels good.

Chapter 1: The Red Light Revolution— What's All the Buzz About?

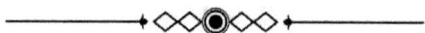

A few years ago, I found myself in a small, windowless room at a recovery clinic in Boulder, Colorado. The specialist had just flipped a switch, bathing the entire space in an intense ruby glow that made everything look as if we had stepped into a darkroom for developing photographs—or perhaps the command deck of a submarine in a 1990s action movie.

"Just stand there for about 10 minutes," she said casually, as if asking me to wait while she fetched the mail.

"That's it?" I asked. "Just... stand here?"

She nodded. "That's it. The light does all the work."

I'll admit, my inner skeptic was having a field day. I had just paid good money to stand in what amounted to a red lightbulb closet. As someone who has spent years researching health interventions, I'm no stranger to wellness trends that promise the moon and deliver a pebble.

However, what happened over the following weeks after regular sessions—improved sleep, faster workout recovery, and a noticeable improvement in an old, nagging shoulder injury—left me both intrigued and slightly embarrassed about my initial judgment.

This is probably a good time to acknowledge that, right now, red light therapy occupies a peculiar position in the wellness landscape. For some, it is already a non-negotiable part of their daily routine, as essential as brushing their teeth or having morning coffee. For others, it still carries the suspicious aura of being "too good to be true" or "just another biohacking fad that Silicon Valley bros are obsessed with."

And honestly? I understand both perspectives.

From Fringe to Mainstream: The Red Light Journey

Red light therapy (RLT)—sometimes called photobiomodulation, low-level laser therapy, or LED light therapy—has actually been around longer than you might think. The concept of using light for healing dates back thousands of years to ancient Egyptian, Greek, and Chinese civilizations, which used sunlight therapeutically. The modern approach began in the 1960s when a Hungarian physician named Endre Mester accidentally discovered that low-power laser light could stimulate hair growth and wound healing in mice.

However, it is only in the last decade that red light therapy has transitioned from an obscure medical treatment to a mainstream wellness practice. You might have first encountered it at a high-end spa, a physical therapist's office, a dermatologist's clinic, or, increasingly, in someone's home bathroom.

The technology has followed the classic innovation curve: First adopted by professional athletes and celebrities with access to expensive, clinical-grade equipment, it has gradually become accessible to everyday wellness enthusiasts as costs decreased and home devices improved. Today, you can find everything from $20 handheld red light devices to $10,000 full-body panels online.

NASA even got involved, using red light therapy to help grow plants in space and later to treat muscle atrophy in astronauts. When NASA takes an interest in something, it is usually a sign that you should pay attention. (Though I should clarify that this does not apply to all space-related innovations—the freeze-dried ice cream they developed is frankly disappointing. Trust me, I have tried it.)

What Makes Red Light Special?

Here's where we need to take a quick detour into the electromagnetic spectrum—don't worry, I promise to keep this short and painless.

Light exists on a spectrum. On one end, you have gamma rays and X-rays, which have very short wavelengths. On the other end, you have radio waves, which have very long wavelengths. Somewhere in the middle is the visible light spectrum—the colors we can see with our eyes.

Red light sits at the beginning of the visible spectrum, with wavelengths between approximately 630 and 700 nanometers (nm). Near-infrared light, which is invisible to our eyes but is often included in red light therapy devices, ranges from about 700 to 1100 nm.

These specific wavelengths turn out to be special because they can penetrate human tissue at different depths. While blue light mostly affects the surface of your skin (which is why it's used for acne treatments), red and near-infrared light can reach much deeper—up to several centimeters into your body.

But depth isn't the only factor that matters. Something even more fascinating happens when these specific wavelengths interact with our cells. They are absorbed by a part of our cells called mitochondria—those little powerhouses you might remember from high school biology class that create energy for everything your body does.

When red and near-infrared light hits these mitochondria, it essentially gives them a boost, like adding a turbocharger to an engine. The mitochondria then produce more energy, function more efficiently, and create beneficial signaling molecules that affect the entire cell.

This increased cellular energy doesn't just make you feel more energetic (though that's one benefit); it also helps cells perform their specialized jobs better. Skin cells can produce more collagen and elastin, muscle cells can repair damage faster, and brain cells can maintain healthier connections.

This is why red light therapy doesn't just have one benefit but seems to help with many different things—it's optimizing a fundamental cellular process that affects your entire body.

What Red Light Therapy Is NOT

Before we go any further, let's clear up some misconceptions about what red light therapy is not because there is plenty of confusion out there.

First, red light therapy is not the same as infrared saunas. While both use parts of the light spectrum to benefit health, they work through completely different mechanisms. Infrared saunas primarily use far-infrared wavelengths (which are much longer than near-infrared) to heat your body directly, causing you to sweat and creating a thermal stress response. Red light therapy does not generate significant heat and works through non-thermal photobiomodulation effects at the cellular level.

Second, red light therapy is not a sunbed or tanning booth. In fact, it is the opposite in many ways. Tanning booths use UV light that damages skin cells to trigger a protective melanin response. Red light therapy uses much longer wavelengths that do not damage cells but instead help them function better.

Third, red light therapy is not a magic cure-all or a replacement for fundamental health practices. No light device will override the effects of poor sleep, terrible nutrition, or chronic stress. Think of red light therapy as an enhancement to a solid foundation, not a miracle that will single-handedly transform your health.

Finally, and I find myself repeating this often, not all red lights are created equal. The holiday lights you put up in December, a red lightbulb from the hardware store, or the red filter on your phone's flashlight do not provide therapeutic benefits. The specific wavelengths, power output, and treatment protocols matter enormously, which is why we will spend an entire chapter discussing devices and how to choose the right one.

The Benefits: What Can Red Light Actually Do?

When I first began researching the benefits of red light therapy, I found myself repeatedly saying, "Wait, it can help with that too?" The research is broad and growing rapidly, with thousands of peer-reviewed studies examining various applications.

Here's a quick overview of the most well-established benefits, which we will explore in depth in Chapter 3:

1. **Pain Relief and Reduced Inflammation:** Red light therapy has been shown to reduce inflammation and provide pain relief for conditions ranging from arthritis to back pain. Unlike pain medications, it addresses underlying inflammation rather than merely masking symptoms.

2. **Skin Health and Anti-Aging:** Perhaps the most visible benefit is improved skin

health—such as increased collagen production, reduced wrinkles, improved tone and texture, and even assistance with conditions like eczema, rosacea, and psoriasis.

3. **Enhanced Energy and Performance:** By improving mitochondrial function, red light therapy can increase energy at the cellular level, thereby enhancing physical performance and reducing fatigue.

4. **Accelerated Recovery:** Athletes and weekend warriors alike report significantly faster recovery from workouts and injuries when using red light therapy.

5. **Improved Sleep Quality:** Regular exposure to red light, particularly in the evening, can help regulate circadian rhythms and melatonin production, leading to better sleep quality.

6. **Hair Growth Stimulation:** Similar to its effects on skin, red light therapy can stimulate hair follicles, aiding in the treatment of thinning hair and certain types of hair loss.

7. **Mood and Cognitive Function:** Emerging research suggests benefits for brain health, cognitive performance, and

even mood disorders such as depression and anxiety.

8. **Metabolic Health:** Some studies indicate benefits for fat loss, especially when combined with exercise, along with improvements in metabolic markers.

What fascinates me most about these benefits is that they are not just subjective improvements that people report feeling—though those exist as well. Many of these benefits have been measured in objective ways: Reduced inflammatory markers in blood tests, increased collagen density in skin biopsies, improved strength and endurance in controlled physical tests, changes in brain wave patterns, and more.

In other words, this is not just a placebo effect at work, though I should note that the placebo effect itself is a powerful phenomenon that should not be dismissed. The benefits of red light therapy have been demonstrated in thousands of double-blind, placebo-controlled studies—the gold standard of scientific research.

Why Hasn't My Doctor Recommended This?

At this point, you might be wondering, "If red light therapy is so beneficial, why hasn't my doctor recommended it?" It's a fair question, and there are several reasons.

First, most conventional medical education provides minimal training in light-based therapies or emerging physical modalities. Medical schools focus heavily on pharmaceutical interventions and surgical techniques, with limited time devoted to preventive approaches or complementary therapies.

Second, the research, while substantial and growing, is scattered across many different specialties. Dermatologists study its effects on the skin, while physical therapists and sports medicine doctors examine its impact on injury recovery. Neurologists investigate its effects on brain health. Few practitioners have the time or incentive to stay current on research outside their specific fields.

Third, until recently, effective red light therapy required expensive, clinical-grade equipment that wasn't practical for most medical offices, let alone home use. This is rapidly changing as technology improves and costs decrease, but many healthcare providers simply aren't aware of these developments.

Finally, there's the challenge of standardization. With pharmaceutical treatments, doctors can prescribe specific dosages with predictable effects. Light therapy has more variables: wavelengths, power output, treatment distance, treatment time, and frequency all matter. Without standardized "prescriptions," many doctors hesitate to make specific recommendations.

This doesn't mean that no medical professionals recommend red light therapy—many forward-thinking practitioners do, and clinical usage is growing. However, it does explain why you might not have heard about it from your primary care physician.

The Personal Journey: Why I Wrote This Book

I've spent the last several years diving deep into the world of red light therapy—not just reading the research, but also connecting with the pioneering scientists conducting it, the clinicians applying it, and, most importantly, the everyday people experiencing its benefits.

What struck me most was the gap between what is known in research circles and what is accessible to regular people who could benefit. Too often, potentially life-changing interventions remain stuck in academic journals or clinical settings, never making it into the hands of those who need them most.

I wrote this book because I believe red light therapy represents one of the most accessible, safe, and effective health tools available today. However, like any tool, its value depends entirely on how you use it.

The 30-day framework I will share in this book has been refined through work with hundreds of individuals across different age groups, health conditions, and fitness levels. It is designed to help you experience measurable benefits within a month while setting you up for sustainable, long-term use.

This isn't about adding another complicated health protocol to your already busy life. It is about finding the minimum effective dose that delivers maximum results and integrating it seamlessly into your existing routine.

In the next chapter, we will dive deeper into the science behind red light therapy—explained in a way that actually makes sense without requiring a biology degree. But first, I want to share a quick exercise that will help you get the most from this 30-day journey.

Your Starting Point: A Quick Self-Assessment

Before beginning any new health practice, it is valuable to establish a clear baseline. This helps you objectively track your progress and notice improvements that might otherwise be too subtle or gradual to detect.

Take a few minutes to rate yourself on a scale of 1 to 10 in the following areas:

- Energy level throughout the day
- Sleep quality and how rested you feel upon waking
- Recovery time after physical activity
- Current pain levels (note specific problem areas)
- Skin health and appearance
- Mood and mental clarity
- Overall sense of vitality

For any areas you rated below a 7, write a brief description of what specific improvements would look like. For example, instead of just noting "poor sleep," you might write, "I want to fall asleep within 15 minutes of going to bed and wake up feeling refreshed without an alarm."

Being specific about your starting point and desired improvements will help you notice the sometimes subtle but meaningful changes that occur as you implement the protocols in this book.

In the next chapter, we will explore exactly how red light therapy works at the cellular level and why these specific wavelengths have such powerful effects on your body. Don't worry—I promise to explain the complex science in a way that not only makes sense but might actually make you excited about mitochondria for the first time in your life.

Chapter 2: The Science Made Simple–
How Red Light Actually Works

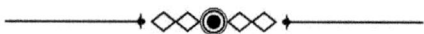

I once watched a three-year-old try to explain how airplanes stay in the sky. "The clouds push them up," she said with absolute certainty. Her explanation was adorable, completely wrong, and yet—surprisingly useful for her purposes. It provided her with enough of a framework to make sense of what she was seeing without requiring an understanding of Bernoulli's principle or the complex physics of lift.

When it comes to red light therapy, most explanations fall into two extremes. Either they are childishly simplistic ("the light makes your cells happy!") or they consist of dense academic papers filled with terms like "cytochrome c oxidase upregulation" and "retrograde mitochondrial signaling." Neither is particularly helpful for most of us.

So let's find the sweet spot: An explanation that is scientifically accurate but doesn't require a Ph.D. to understand. I promise not to insult your intelligence or overwhelm you with jargon. My goal is simple—by the end of this chapter, you will understand enough about how red light therapy works to use it effectively and explain it confidently to others.

The Light Spectrum: Not All Colors Are Created Equal

Let's start with the basics. Light exists on a spectrum, ranging from very short wavelengths (gamma rays, X-rays) to very long wavelengths (radio waves, microwaves). The visible light spectrum—the colors we can see—occupies just a tiny slice of this range, from about 380 nm (violet) to 700 nm (red).

Red light therapy primarily uses two specific ranges of wavelengths:

- **Red light:** 630–660 nm (visible)
- **Near-infrared light:** 810–850 nm (invisible to the human eye).

These specific wavelengths are not chosen arbitrarily; they represent what scientists call the "optical window" or "therapeutic window," where light can penetrate human tissue effectively and trigger beneficial biological responses.

Shorter wavelengths (like blue light) can only penetrate the surface of the skin. Much longer wavelengths (like far-infrared) mostly create heat. However, red and near-infrared light hit a sweet spot where they can reach deeper tissues without generating significant heat or causing damage.

Think of it like this: if you shine a flashlight through your hand in a dark room, you'll notice a red glow on the other side. That's because red light can travel through tissue, while other colors (like blue or green) get completely absorbed or scattered. This simple observation reveals something profound about how different wavelengths interact with our bodies.

The Mitochondria Connection: Cellular Power Plants

Now let's talk about what happens when these specific wavelengths reach your cells. The key player in this story is an often-overlooked cellular component: the mitochondrion (mitochondria in the plural).

You might vaguely remember mitochondria from high school biology—they are often described as the "powerhouses of the cell." This is actually a pretty good description. Mitochondria take the food we eat and the oxygen we breathe and convert them into a form of energy our cells can use, called ATP (adenosine triphosphate).

ATP is essentially the energy currency of your cells. Every process in your body that requires energy—from muscle contraction to brain function to cellular repair—depends on ATP. The more efficiently your mitochondria produce ATP, the better your cells function.

Here's where red light enters the picture. Inside your mitochondria is an enzyme called cytochrome c oxidase (CCO). This enzyme plays a crucial role in the final step of ATP production. And here is the key insight: CCO strongly absorbs red and near-infrared light.

When CCO absorbs these specific wavelengths, it becomes more active and efficient. This leads to several interrelated effects:

1. **Increased ATP production:** Your cellular powerhouses make more energy.

2. **Enhanced mitochondrial function:** The entire energy production system works more efficiently.

3. **Release of nitric oxide:** A signaling molecule that improves blood flow and cellular communication.

4. **Creation of reactive oxygen species (ROS):** In small, controlled amounts, these act as signaling molecules that trigger protective and regenerative mechanisms.

This boost in cellular energy doesn't just make your cells "happier;" it enhances their ability to perform specific functions. Skin cells can produce more collagen and elastin, muscle cells can contract more efficiently and repair damage faster, brain cells can maintain healthier neural connections, and immune cells can better fight infections and resolve inflammation.

Beyond Mitochondria: The Ripple Effects

The mitochondrial effects I just described are the primary mechanism of red light therapy, but they trigger a cascade of secondary effects throughout your body. Let me highlight a few of these downstream benefits:

Improved Circulation and Blood Flow

When red light stimulates the release of nitric oxide (a vasodilator), blood vessels expand, increasing blood flow to tissues. This brings more oxygen and nutrients to cells while removing waste products more efficiently. The result is faster healing, reduced inflammation, and improved cellular function.

This effect is easily visible if you examine infrared images of the body before and after red light therapy; treated areas show increased heat signatures as blood flow increases to those regions.

Reduced Oxidative Stress

While excessive free radicals (reactive oxygen species) can damage cells, the small, controlled amounts created during red light therapy actually trigger protective responses. It's similar to how exercise creates short-term stress that leads to long-term resilience.

Red light therapy activates your body's natural antioxidant defense systems, including superoxide dismutase (SOD) and glutathione peroxidase. These systems help neutralize damaging free radicals throughout your body, not just in the treated area.

Modulated Inflammatory Response

Inflammation has become something of a boogeyman in health discussions, but it's important to remember that inflammation itself isn't inherently bad—it's a crucial part of your body's healing process. The problem occurs when inflammation becomes chronic or excessive.

Red light therapy doesn't simply "reduce inflammation" in a blunt way. Instead, it helps normalize the inflammatory response: enhancing acute inflammation when needed for healing while helping to resolve chronic inflammation that is no longer serving a purpose.

Cellular Signaling and Gene Expression

Perhaps the most fascinating effects of red light therapy occur at the level of gene expression. When cells are exposed to specific wavelengths of red and near-infrared light, they change the expression of genes related to:

- Collagen and elastin production
- Cell proliferation and growth
- Antioxidant response
- Anti-inflammatory mediators
- Cell survival and apoptosis (programmed cell death)

These changes in gene expression help explain why the benefits of red light therapy can continue for days after a treatment session and why consistent use leads to cumulative improvements over time.

Different Wavelengths, Different Benefits

I mentioned earlier that red light therapy typically uses two distinct ranges of wavelengths: visible red light (630–660 nm) and near-infrared light (810–850 nm). These different wavelengths have somewhat different effects due to their penetration depth and the cellular components they influence.

Red light (630–660 nm) penetrates tissue to a depth of about 8–10 mm. This makes it ideal for:

- Skin conditions
- Superficial wound healing
- Hair follicle stimulation
- Surface inflammation

Near-infrared light (810–850 nm) can penetrate much deeper, potentially reaching 30–50 mm into the body. This makes it more effective for:

- Deep tissue injuries
- Joint pain and inflammation
- Muscle recovery
- Bone healing
- Brain health (through the skull)

Many high-quality red light therapy devices include both wavelength ranges to provide maximum benefits. The visible red wavelengths address surface issues, while the invisible near-infrared wavelengths penetrate deeper tissues.

What the Research Actually Shows

The scientific literature on red light therapy is vast and growing rapidly. A search on PubMed (the main database for biomedical research) for terms related to red light therapy returns over 7,000 peer-reviewed studies, with hundreds of new papers published each year.

These studies range from cellular research in Petri dishes to animal models to human clinical trials. They cover applications as diverse as wound healing, pain management, cognitive function, athletic performance, and skin rejuvenation.

While the quality of research varies (as with any field), there is a substantial body of high-quality evidence supporting specific applications of red light therapy. Some of the strongest evidence exists for:

- **Pain reduction:** Multiple meta-analyses (studies that combine results from many individual studies) show significant pain relief for conditions such as osteoarthritis, neck pain, and low back pain.

- **Wound healing:** Both diabetic ulcers and surgical wounds have been shown to heal faster with appropriate red light therapy protocols.

- **Skin rejuvenation:** Increases in collagen production, improved skin tone and texture, and reduced wrinkles have been demonstrated in controlled trials.

- **Hair regrowth:** For certain types of hair loss, particularly androgenetic alopecia, red light therapy has shown promising results.

- **Muscle recovery:** Several well-designed studies indicate faster recovery and reduced muscle soreness after exercise when red light therapy is applied.

I'll dive deeper into specific benefits in the next chapter, but the important point here is that red light therapy isn't just supported by anecdotal evidence or theoretical mechanisms—there is substantial clinical research backing it up.

Dose Matters: The Biphasic Dose Response

One of the most critical concepts to understand about red light therapy is something called the "biphasic dose response." This principle explains why more isn't always better when it comes to light exposure.

The biphasic dose response means that benefits increase as the dose increases—but only up to a point. After that optimal point, more exposure actually provides fewer benefits or could even cause negative effects.

This creates what scientists call an "inverted U-shaped curve" of benefits. Too little light, and you won't see results. Too much light, and you might inhibit the very processes you're trying to stimulate.

This principle explains why some people don't see benefits from red light therapy—they are either undertreating (using devices with insufficient power output or treating for too short a time) or overtreating (using high-powered devices for too long or treating too frequently).

Getting the dose right involves balancing several factors:

- Wavelength (nm)
- Power density (mW/cm^2)
- Treatment time (seconds/minutes)
- Treatment frequency (daily, every other day, etc.)
- Distance from the device

- Area being treated

Don't worry if this sounds complicated—in Chapter 5, I will provide specific protocols that take all these factors into account, giving you clear guidance on exactly what to do to achieve your specific goals.

Common Misconceptions About Red Light Therapy

Before we wrap up this chapter, let's address some common misconceptions about red light therapy:

Misconception #1: "Red light therapy is just a placebo effect."

While placebo effects are real and powerful, red light therapy has been shown to create measurable physiological changes in controlled studies, including effects on cell cultures where placebo effects are not possible. These changes include increased ATP production, alterations in gene expression, increased collagen synthesis, and modified inflammatory markers.

Misconception #2: "Any red light will work."

The specific wavelengths, power density, and treatment parameters matter significantly. A standard red LED lightbulb, a heat lamp with a red filter, or the red setting on a flashlight will not provide therapeutic benefits. Effective devices must deliver the correct wavelengths (630–660 nm and/or 810–850 nm) at sufficient power density.

Misconception #3: "Red light therapy is dangerous for the eyes."

While you should follow safety guidelines for any light-based therapy, red and near-infrared wavelengths are actually among the safest parts of the light spectrum for eye exposure. Unlike UV light or blue light, which can damage retinal cells, red and near-infrared light at therapeutic intensities has been shown to be safe and potentially beneficial for eye health. That said, very bright light of any wavelength can be uncomfortable, so many users prefer to close their eyes or wear appropriate eyewear during treatments.

Misconception #4: "You need expensive professional equipment to see benefits."

While professional-grade devices do offer advantages in terms of power output and treatment area, there are now many affordable home devices that can provide therapeutic benefits when used correctly. The key is understanding the specifications and using appropriate treatment protocols.

Misconception #5: "Red light therapy works instantly."

Some benefits, such as increased circulation and reduced muscle soreness, may be noticeable after a single session. However, most significant benefits develop over time with consistent use, typically over weeks or months. Like exercise or good nutrition, red light therapy works best as a consistent practice rather than as a one-time treatment.

Putting It All Together: A Simple Explanation

To summarize everything, we've covered in plain language:

Red light therapy works by delivering specific wavelengths of red and near-infrared light that penetrate your skin and reach your cells. These wavelengths are absorbed by your mitochondria (the cellular power plants), which respond by producing more energy, functioning more efficiently, and triggering a cascade of beneficial effects throughout your body.

These effects include increased circulation, reduced inflammation, enhanced cellular repair, and changes in gene expression that support healing and regeneration. Different wavelengths penetrate to different depths, allowing for the treatment of both surface issues and deeper tissues.

Like any effective therapy, the dose matters—too little won't help, and too much may hinder progress. The research supporting red light therapy is substantial and growing, with particularly strong evidence for pain relief, skin health, wound healing, and recovery from exercise.

In the next chapter, we'll explore the specific benefits of red light therapy in greater detail, examining what the science says about each application and what kind of results you can realistically expect. Then, in later chapters, we'll delve into the practical aspects of choosing devices and implementing effective treatment protocols.

For now, I hope you have a clearer understanding of how this remarkable therapy actually works—no Ph.D. required.

Chapter 3: The Health Revolution– Benefits Beyond the Hype

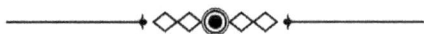

———— ✦◇◇◉◇◇✦ ————

When I first began exploring red light therapy, I felt that familiar skepticism we all develop after seeing too many "miracle cure" headlines. You know the feeling—that internal eye roll when someone claims their new wellness practice is going to solve every health problem, from hangnails to existential dread.

So, it came as a genuine surprise when I kept encountering serious researchers, clinicians, and everyday users who weren't just moderately impressed with red light therapy; they were downright enthusiastic. And not in that vague, "I feel better somehow" way, but in specific, measurable ways backed by before-and-after photos, lab tests, and clinical studies.

In this chapter, we're going to explore what red light therapy can really do—beyond both the dismissive skepticism and the over-the-top hype. I'll share the benefits that have the strongest scientific support, explain what results you can realistically expect, and provide examples of real people experiencing these benefits.

But first, an important caveat: No health intervention works for everyone. Despite what some overzealous marketers might claim, red light therapy isn't going to transform every aspect of your health overnight. What it can do, when used correctly, is provide meaningful improvements across several dimensions of health and well-being. Let's explore what those are.

Pain Relief and Inflammation Reduction

If there is one benefit of red light therapy with overwhelming scientific support, it is pain relief. This is not just subjective reporting; numerous controlled clinical trials have demonstrated significant reductions in pain scores and objective measures of inflammation.

The mechanisms behind this pain relief are multifaceted:

1. **Reduced inflammation:** Red and near-infrared light modulate inflammatory processes, reducing pro-inflammatory cytokines while supporting the resolution phase of inflammation.

2. **Improved circulation:** By stimulating nitric oxide release, red light therapy enhances blood flow to damaged tissues, bringing in healing nutrients and removing inflammatory waste products.

3. **Nerve modulation:** These wavelengths can temporarily reduce the excitability of pain-transmitting nerves, providing immediate relief similar to how cold therapy works.

4. **Accelerated tissue repair:** By enhancing cellular energy production, red light therapy speeds up the repair of damaged tissues that may be causing pain.

The research is particularly strong for certain types of pain:

Joint Pain and Arthritis: Multiple studies have shown that red light therapy can reduce pain and improve function in both rheumatoid arthritis and osteoarthritis. A meta-analysis of 22 randomized controlled trials concluded that red light therapy significantly reduced pain in patients with knee osteoarthritis and improved their functional ability.

Low Back Pain: Several well-designed studies have demonstrated meaningful pain reduction for chronic low back pain. One particularly compelling study found that just seven sessions of red light therapy provided a 50% reduction in pain that persisted for months after the treatment ended.

What makes red light therapy particularly valuable for pain management is that, unlike many pharmaceutical approaches, it addresses underlying causes rather than merely masking symptoms. It is also remarkably free of side effects when used correctly.

Skin Health and Anti-Aging

The skin benefits of red light therapy are perhaps the most visibly obvious and well-documented. When I surveyed users about the results they noticed first, improved skin consistently topped the list.

Here's what the research shows red light therapy can do for the skin:

- **Increased Collagen Production:** Multiple studies have shown that red light therapy increases collagen production. One study found a 31% increase in collagen density after 12 weeks of red light treatment.

- **Reduced Wrinkles and Fine Lines:** Research published in Photomedicine and Laser Surgery found significant improvements in skin complexion, skin tone, and wrinkle reduction after red light therapy treatments.

- **Improved Complexion and Tone:** Red light therapy has been shown to improve skin tone, reduce redness, and create a more even complexion by promoting healthy cellular function and reducing inflammation.

- **Accelerated Wound Healing:** For cuts, scrapes, burns, or surgical incisions, red light therapy has been shown to speed healing by an average of 40% in multiple studies.

- **Help with Skin Conditions:** Red light therapy has shown benefits for conditions including psoriasis, eczema, rosacea, adult acne, and scarring.

What makes red light therapy particularly unique for skin health is that it works from the inside out, stimulating your skin's natural regenerative processes rather than just treating surface symptoms.

Enhanced Energy and Performance

Fatigue and low energy are among the most common complaints that people bring to healthcare providers. While there are many potential causes, issues with cellular energy production underlie many cases of persistent fatigue.

The research on red light therapy for energy enhancement shows several important benefits:

- **Increased Cellular Energy Production:** By stimulating the enzyme cytochrome c oxidase, red light therapy enhances the production of ATP (adenosine triphosphate), the primary energy currency of our cells. Studies using muscle biopsies before and after red light therapy have shown increases in ATP production of up to 200% in treated tissues.

- **Improved Exercise Performance:** Multiple studies have demonstrated that pre-exercise red light therapy can enhance physical performance. A meta-analysis of 46 clinical trials found that red light therapy before exercise consistently improved performance measures, including increased time to exhaustion, greater total work performed, and reduced perceived exertion.

- **Reduced Fatigue:** For those dealing with chronic fatigue, several studies have shown promise. One study of patients with fibromyalgia found significant reductions in fatigue levels, along with improved sleep quality, after 10 sessions of red light therapy.

The energy-enhancing effects of red light therapy tend to be cumulative, with many users reporting that the benefits build over weeks of consistent use.

Accelerated Recovery and Healing

One of the most valued benefits among athletes and fitness enthusiasts is red light therapy's ability to speed up recovery and reduce soreness after intense physical activity.

Research shows several mechanisms by which red light therapy enhances recovery:

- **Reduced Delayed-Onset Muscle Soreness (DOMS):** Multiple studies have shown that red light therapy, when administered before or after exercise, can significantly reduce the severity and duration of muscle soreness. A randomized controlled trial found that participants who received red light therapy immediately after intense eccentric exercise experienced 35% less muscle soreness at 48 hours compared to the control group.

- **Accelerated Muscle Repair:** When muscles are damaged during exercise, red light therapy appears to accelerate the repair process by enhancing protein synthesis and reducing oxidative stress.

- **Faster Tendon and Ligament Healing:** For common soft tissue injuries, such as tendonitis or ligament sprains, red light therapy has been shown to speed up healing by improving collagen synthesis and alignment.

Many professional sports teams and Olympic training centers now incorporate red light therapy into their recovery protocols, reporting significant improvements in recovery times and reduced injury rates among their athletes.

Improved Sleep Quality

Sleep issues affect an estimated 50 to 70 million Americans, with wide-ranging impacts on health, cognition, and quality of life. Red light therapy has shown promising results for improving sleep quality through several mechanisms:

- **Circadian Rhythm Regulation:** Unlike blue light, which suppresses melatonin production, red wavelengths do not interfere with melatonin and may help establish stronger circadian cues when used in the evening.

- **Enhanced Melatonin Production:** Some studies suggest that red light exposure may actively support natural melatonin production, thereby improving the body's natural sleep signals.

- **Reduced Cortisol and Stress Response:** Evening red light therapy sessions have been shown to reduce cortisol levels and activate parasympathetic nervous system responses, helping the body transition into a more relaxed state conducive to sleep.

A study published in the Journal of Athletic Training found that red light therapy not only improved subjective sleep quality in basketball players but also enhanced melatonin levels, reduced cortisol, and led to better athletic performance the following day.

Hair Growth Stimulation

Hair loss affects millions of people and can significantly impact self-esteem and quality of life. Red light therapy has emerged as a promising non-pharmaceutical approach for certain types of hair loss, particularly androgenetic alopecia (pattern baldness) in both men and women.

The research on red light therapy for hair growth shows several mechanisms of action:

- **Increased Blood Flow to Follicles:** By stimulating nitric oxide release and vasodilation, red light therapy enhances blood flow to hair follicles, delivering more nutrients and oxygen to support healthy hair growth.

- **Extended Growth Phase:** Hair grows in cycles, with phases of growth (anagen), transition (catagen), and rest (telogen). Red light therapy appears to extend the growth phase, allowing hairs to grow longer and thicker before transitioning to the resting phase.

The evidence for red light therapy's effectiveness in promoting hair growth is substantial enough that the FDA has cleared several red light devices specifically for treating androgenetic alopecia. Results typically take time to become visible; most studies show initial results at 3 to 4 months, with maximum benefits observed at 6 to 12 months of consistent use.

Cognitive Function and Brain Health

One of the most exciting emerging areas of red light therapy research involves its effects on brain function. While this field is newer than some other applications, the preliminary research is promising.

The research on red light therapy for cognitive function shows several potential benefits:

- **Improved Cerebral Blood Flow:** Near-infrared light can penetrate the skull and enhance blood flow to the brain, delivering more oxygen and nutrients to brain cells.

- **Enhanced Mitochondrial Function in Neurons:** Brain cells have high-energy demands, and the mitochondrial support provided by red light therapy may help them function more efficiently.

- **Reduced Neuroinflammation:** Chronic inflammation in the brain contributes to cognitive decline and is implicated in neurodegenerative conditions. The anti-inflammatory effects of red light therapy may help create a healthier brain environment.

A study from the University of California found that a single 15-minute session of transcranial near-infrared light improved attention, memory, and executive function in healthy adults. The effects were measurable immediately after treatment.

What Can You Realistically Expect?

With all these potential benefits, you might be wondering what you can personally expect from incorporating red light therapy into your routine. While individual responses vary, here is a realistic timeline of benefits that many users experience:

First Week (1–7 Days)

- Improved skin appearance (often a subtle "glow" as circulation improves)
- Reduced pain in treated areas (temporary relief that builds with consistency)
- Enhanced recovery after workouts (reduced muscle soreness)
- Improved sleep quality (particularly if used in evening sessions)

First Month (8–30 Days)

- More noticeable skin improvements (tone, texture, and minor blemish reduction)
- Longer-lasting pain relief
- More consistent energy levels

- Continued improvements in sleep quality and duration
- Initial signs of hair thickening (for those using it for hair growth)

Second and Third Months (31–90 Days)

- Significant improvements in skin elasticity and collagen density
- Substantial reduction in chronic pain for many users
- Measurable improvements in wound healing and recovery times
- Noticeable hair growth in previously thinning areas
- More stable energy and mood

A few important points to remember:

1. **Consistency matters more than intensity:** Regular sessions according to proper protocols yield better results than occasional high-intensity treatments.

2. **Benefits are cumulative:** Many of the effects of red light therapy build over time as cellular function improves and tissues regenerate.

3. **Individual responses vary:** Factors such as age, baseline health status, specific

conditions, and concurrent health practices all influence your results.

4. **Red light therapy works best as part of a comprehensive approach:** While it can provide standalone benefits, the most impressive results occur when combined with proper nutrition, adequate sleep, stress management, and appropriate physical activity.

When Red Light Therapy Might Not Be the Answer

While red light therapy offers impressive benefits for many conditions, it is not a universal solution for all health concerns. Here are some situations where other interventions may be more appropriate:

- **Acute Injuries:** For fresh injuries with significant swelling and inflammation, cold therapy is often a better first-line approach, with red light therapy potentially introduced during the recovery phase.

- **Serious Medical Conditions:** Red light therapy is a complementary approach, not a replacement for necessary medical treatment of serious conditions. It may support overall health during treatment but should not delay appropriate medical care.

In the next chapter, we will dive into practical considerations for choosing the right red light therapy device for your specific needs and budget. After all, even the most powerful therapy is only effective if you can access it consistently and use it correctly.

Chapter 4: Your Red Light Toolkit—
Choosing the Right Device

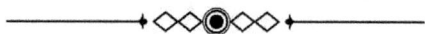

———— ✦ ◇◇◉◇◇ ✦ ————

The first time I went shopping for a red light therapy device, I felt as if I were trying to buy a car without knowing how to drive. The terminology was unfamiliar, the price range was bewildering (ranging from $30 to over $10,000), and every manufacturer claimed that their device was revolutionary. I ended up making an expensive mistake—purchasing a device that looked impressive but delivered such a low-power output that it was practically useless for anything beyond illuminating my bathroom with a red glow.

I don't want you to waste your money or time on ineffective devices. In this chapter, I will demystify red light therapy technology and provide you with a clear framework for choosing the right device for your specific needs and budget. We will cover which features actually matter, which specifications to pay attention to, and how to see through marketing hype to find devices that deliver real results.

Understanding the Key Specifications

Before we look at different types of devices, let's establish the critical specifications that determine whether a device will be effective:

Wavelength

As we discussed in Chapter 2, therapeutic red light falls into two main ranges:

- **Red light:** 630–660 nanometers (nm)
- Near-infrared (NIR) light: 810–850 nm

The best devices offer both ranges, as they penetrate to different depths and provide complementary benefits. Red wavelengths work well for surface concerns, such as skin health and superficial pain, while near-infrared light penetrates deeper for muscle recovery, joint pain, and internal benefits.

Be wary of devices that do not clearly specify their exact wavelengths or use vague terms like "multiple wavelengths across the spectrum." Effective devices typically utilize narrowband wavelengths centered around specific peaks (often 660 nm and 850 nm) rather than a broad spectrum of light.

Power Output and Irradiance

This is where many inexpensive devices fall short. Power output determines how much light energy actually reaches your tissues—and, thus, whether you will see results.

Power output is typically measured in two ways:

- **Total output** (in watts): The overall power the device produces.

- **Irradiance** (in mW/cm^2): The power density per square centimeter at a specific distance.

Irradiance is the more important measure because it indicates how much power is actually delivered to your tissues. Clinical studies typically use irradiance levels between 20 and 100 mW/cm^2 at the treatment surface.

Many budget devices advertise impressive-sounding total output numbers but deliver very low irradiance. For example, a device might claim "300 watts of power!" but deliver only 5 to 110 mW/cm^2 at the recommended treatment distance—far below the therapeutic threshold established in research.

Treatment Area

The size of the device determines how much of your body can be treated at once, which affects both treatment time and convenience:

- **Small targeted devices** (handheld or small panels): Good for treating specific problem areas, such as the face, joints, or small pain sites.

- **Medium panels** (approximately 12" x 6" to 24" x 12"): Suitable for treating larger areas, such as the back, chest, or legs, one section at a time.

- **Large panels or full-body systems:** Allow for the treatment of large portions of the body simultaneously, reducing total treatment time.

If you're primarily interested in facial rejuvenation or treating a specific joint, a smaller device may suffice. For whole-body benefits or treating multiple areas, larger panels or modular systems that can be expanded over time are more practical.

LED Quality and Lens Angle

The quality of LEDs and their lens design significantly impact a device's effectiveness:

- **LED quality:** Medical-grade LEDs from reputable manufacturers deliver more consistent wavelengths and last longer.

- **Lens angle:** This determines how focused the light is; narrower angles (typically 30-60 degrees) deliver more concentrated light with less scatter.

Better devices use high-quality LEDs with optical lenses that focus the light appropriately for therapeutic use. Budget devices often use cheap LEDs with wide-angle dispersion (90-120 degrees), meaning much of the light scatters rather than penetrating tissue.

EMF Levels

Electromagnetic field (EMF) emissions are a concern for some users, especially with the daily use of electrical devices close to the body. Quality red light therapy devices should have low EMF levels, ideally below 2 milligauss at the treatment distance.

Reputable manufacturers will provide EMF testing information. If a company does not address EMF concerns or provide testing data, it may be a red flag regarding their overall quality standards.

Types of Red Light Therapy Devices

Now that we understand the critical specifications, let's explore the main categories of devices available:

1. Handheld Devices

Price range: $30–$300

Pros

- Most affordable entry point
- Portable and convenient for travel
- Good for targeted treatment of small areas (face, joints, small pain sites)
- Easy to position at different angles

Cons

- Small treatment area means long treatment times for whole-body benefits
- Often have lower power output than larger panels
- Many inexpensive models have insufficient irradiance for clinical results

- Battery life can be limiting in cordless models

Best for: Beginners wanting to test red light therapy without a large investment, travelers, or those focusing only on facial rejuvenation or very targeted treatment of specific small areas.

What to look for: At minimum, 20 mW/cm² irradiance at the recommended treatment distance, clearly specified wavelengths (ideally both red and NIR options), and a treatment area appropriate for your primary use case.

2. Masks and Contoured Devices

Price range: $100–$900

Pros

- Shaped to fit specific body parts (face, neck, knee, etc.)
- Hands-free operation
- Consistent treatment distance across the target area
- Often include both red and NIR wavelengths

Cons

- Only treat specific body areas

- Limited flexibility for different applications
- Quality and power output vary dramatically between products
- Some designs have poor light distribution

Best for: Those with specific treatment targets (like facial rejuvenation or knee pain) who want a dedicated, convenient solution for that area.

What to look for: Even light distribution across the treatment surface, comfortable design for extended sessions, and adequate power output (many mask-style devices have very low irradiance despite high prices).

3. Small to Medium Panels

Price range: $300–$800

Pros

- Larger treatment area than handheld devices
- More powerful than most handheld options
- Versatile for different body areas
- Often represent the best value for most users
- Many include both red and NIR wavelengths

Cons

- Still require multiple sessions to treat the whole body
- Less portable than handheld devices
- Quality and specifications vary widely between brands

Best for: Most home users seeking a balance of versatility, power, and value; athletes focused on recovery; and those treating multiple body areas.

What to look for: Irradiance of at least 30–50 mW/cm² at the recommended treatment distance, even light distribution, low EMF levels, and cooling systems for longer session duration.

4. Large Panels and Full-Body Systems

Price range: $800–$10,000+

Pros

- Treat large body areas simultaneously
- Highest power output and most efficient treatment times
- Most durable construction
- Often feature advanced cooling systems for sustained operation

- Usually feature both red and NIR wavelengths with independent control

Cons

- Significant investment
- Require dedicated space in your home
- Less portable
- May have higher electricity costs with regular use

Best for: Serious biohackers, individuals with chronic pain conditions requiring whole-body treatment, professional settings, families sharing a device, or users seeking maximum convenience and efficiency.

What to look for: Commercial-grade construction, advanced cooling systems, independent control of wavelengths, modular expansion options, irradiance of 50+ mW/cm² at the recommended treatment distance, and low EMF emissions despite the larger size.

Price vs. Value: What's Actually Worth Paying For

One of the most confusing aspects of shopping for red light therapy devices is the enormous price range. Let me break down what additional investments actually get you:

- **$30–$100 Range (Basic Handheld Devices):** Most devices in this range have insufficient power output for clinical benefits, despite marketing claims. They might create a subtle warming sensation and a red glow but rarely deliver meaningful therapeutic effects. They typically have lower-quality LEDs, minimal warranty protection, and limited durability.

- **$100–$300 Range (Better Handheld and Basic Mask Devices):** In this range, you can find some legitimately therapeutic devices with sufficient power output for targeted treatment of small areas. The best devices in this category can be effective for facial rejuvenation and for treating specific small pain sites, though treatment times may be longer compared to more powerful options.

- **$300–$800 Range (Quality Small/Medium Panels):** This is the sweet spot for most individual users, offering sufficient power output, treatment area, and build quality for effective therapy. Devices in this range typically feature both red and

NIR wavelengths, even light distribution, and adequate cooling systems for longer sessions. They represent the best value for most home users.

- **$800–$2,000 Range (Premium Medium and Large Panels):** Devices in this range offer enhanced convenience through larger treatment areas, higher power output for shorter sessions, better cooling systems, and more durable construction. The premium price often includes better warranty protection, customer support, and more sophisticated control options.

- **$2,000+ Range (Professional and Full-Body Systems):** These systems are designed for clinical settings, professional athletes, or serious biohackers. The investment provides maximum treatment area, highest power output, most durable construction, and comprehensive warranty coverage. While expensive, they can be cost-effective for practitioners treating multiple clients or for families sharing a device.

- **My Personal Recommendation:** For most individual users, I recommend starting with a quality device in the $300–$600 range from a reputable manufacturer. This investment provides sufficient power output and treatment area for effective therapy without breaking the bank. If you experience benefits and want to expand, you can always add additional panels or upgrade to a larger system later.

Red Flags: Marketing Claims to Be Wary Of

The red light therapy market is unfortunately filled with exaggerated claims and misleading specifications. Here are some red flags to watch for:

- **"NASA-Approved" or "NASA-Developed" Technology:** While NASA has indeed conducted research on light therapy, they do not endorse or approve specific consumer products. Companies that use NASA logos or claim NASA approval are typically being deceptive.

- **Unrealistic Benefit Claims:** Be suspicious of devices that promise to cure serious medical conditions, deliver overnight transformations, or resolve complex health issues with minimal use. Legitimate red light therapy provides meaningful benefits, but overpromising is a warning sign.

- **Vague or Missing Specifications:**
  Reputable companies clearly state their
  wavelengths, power output, and irradiance
  at specific treatment distances. If a
  company does not provide these details or
  uses vague terms like "high power" without
  numbers, be skeptical.

- **Confusing Power Metrics:** Some
  companies list the "equivalent wattage" of
  their LEDs rather than the actual power
  output, or they might list the total electrical
  consumption instead of the light energy
  delivered. Look for clear irradiance
  specifications (mW/cm^2) at specific
  treatment distances.

- **Too-Good-To-Be-True Pricing:** If a
  device claims to offer the same
  specifications as premium models at a
  fraction of the price, it is likely either
  misrepresenting its specifications or using
  components that will not last. Quality
  LEDs, proper power supplies, and effective
  cooling systems have real costs.

DIY Options: Can You Build Your Own?

For the technically inclined or budget-conscious,
building a DIY red light therapy device is possible.

Several online communities share plans and parts lists for creating everything from small, targeted devices to larger panels.

Potential advantages

- Cost savings (typically 40–60% less than commercial options)
- Customization to your specific needs
- Learning experience about the technology

Important considerations

- Safety must be the top priority (proper electrical components and heat management)
- Sourcing quality LEDs with precise wavelengths can be challenging
- DIY projects rarely look as polished as commercial options
- No warranty protection or customer support

Making Your Decision: A Step-by-Step Approach

With so many factors to consider, here is a practical approach to selecting your device:

Step 1: Define Your Primary Goals

- Are you focusing on skin rejuvenation, pain relief, recovery, sleep improvement, or general health?
- Which body areas will you primarily treat?
- Are you treating a specific condition or seeking general wellness benefits?

Step 2: Determine Your Practical Requirements

- What is your budget (both initial and potential for future expansion)?
- How much space can you dedicate to the device?
- How much time can you realistically commit to treatment sessions?
- Will you travel with the device, or will you use it in one location?

Step 3: Identify the Minimum Effective Specifications

- For your primary goals, which wavelengths are most beneficial?

- What irradiance level is needed based on research for your specific applications?

- What treatment area size makes sense for your needs?

Step 4: Research and Compare Options

- Create a shortlist of devices that meet your minimum specifications.

- Compare prices, warranty coverage, and customer support.

- Read reviews from verified purchasers (not just testimonials on manufacturer websites).

- Look for before-and-after results for conditions similar to yours.

Step 5: Make Your Selection with Confidence—With this methodical approach, you can select a device that meets your needs without overspending on unnecessary features or underspending on critical specifications.

Conclusion: Investment in Long-Term Health

I view red light therapy devices as tools for health sovereignty; they allow you to address multiple dimensions of health from the comfort of your home, without ongoing costs beyond the initial investment and minimal electricity usage.

When viewed through this lens, even more expensive devices can represent remarkable value. A quality device might cost between $500 and $1,000 upfront but can provide daily treatments for years—potentially replacing or reducing the need for other interventions that incur ongoing costs.

In the next chapter, we will explore exactly how to use your device with specific protocols for different conditions and goals. After all, even the best device is only effective when used correctly and consistently.

Chapter 5: The Perfect Protocol– Timing, Distance, and Frequency

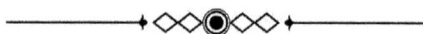

———————◆◇◇◉◇◇◆———————

I once received an email from someone who had purchased an expensive red light therapy device but was seeing no results after six weeks of use. When I asked about their protocol, they told me they were using the device for three minutes a day at arm's length while scrolling through emails on their phone. No wonder they weren't seeing benefits— it's like buying a high-end treadmill but only stepping on it for thirty seconds a day while wearing dress shoes.

In this chapter, we are focusing on what might be the most crucial aspect of red light therapy: How to actually use your device to achieve results. The perfect device is useless without the right protocol, while even a modest device can deliver impressive benefits when used optimally.

Let's break down the essential elements of effective red light therapy protocols and create a practical framework that you can adapt for your specific goals.

The Critical Variables: Creating Your Personal Protocol

Effective red light therapy comes down to five key variables:

1. **Distance:** How far the device is from your body.
2. **Duration:** How long each treatment session lasts.
3. **Frequency:** How often you use the device (daily, every other day, etc.)
4. **Coverage:** Which body areas you treat and in what order.
5. **Timing:** When you use the device relative to other activities and time of day.

Let's explore each of these variables to understand how they work together to create effective protocols.

Distance: Finding the Sweet Spot

The distance between your device and your body dramatically affects the amount of light energy that reaches your tissues. This follows the inverse square law of light: As the distance doubles, the intensity decreases by a factor of four. This means that moving from 6 inches to 12 inches doesn't just halve the intensity; it reduces it to one-quarter of the original power.

Most red light therapy devices are designed to be used at a specific distance, typically:

- Small handheld devices: 0–2 inches
- Masks and contoured devices: Contact or near contact
- Small/medium panels: 6–12 inches
- Large panels: 6–18 inches

The manufacturer's recommended distance is usually based on the device's irradiance (power density) and the target range for therapeutic benefits, typically 20–100 mW/cm^2.

How to determine your optimal distance:

1. **Check manufacturer recommendations:** Start with the distance specified by the manufacturer, as this is typically based on the device's optical design.

2. **Adjust based on comfort:** You should feel gentle warmth but no burning or discomfort. If the device feels too hot, increase the distance slightly.

3. **Consider your goal:** For deeper tissue targets (like muscle recovery or joint pain), you may need to be closer to the device

than for surface treatments like skin rejuvenation.

4. **Be consistent:** Once you find an effective distance, maintain it consistently for better results tracking. Some users mark their ideal distance on the floor or use positioning tools to ensure consistency.

For most home devices, a good starting point is:

- 6–8 inches for red wavelengths (630–660 nm)

- 4–6 inches for near-infrared wavelengths (810–850 nm), which can penetrate deeper tissues even at greater distances

Duration: How Long Is Enough?

Treatment duration depends on several factors, including your device's power output, the condition being treated, and your individual response. However, we can establish some evidence-based guidelines:

For moderate-power devices (30–50 mW/cm²)

- **Minimum effective time:** 5–10 minutes per treatment area

- Optimal range for most applications: 10–20 minutes per treatment area

- **Extended sessions for specific conditions:** 20–30 minutes for chronic or deep-tissue issues

For higher-power devices (50+ mW/cm²)

- **Minimum effective time:** 3–5 minutes per treatment area

- Optimal range for most applications: 5–15 minutes per treatment area

- **Extended sessions for specific conditions:** 15–20 minutes for chronic or deep-tissue issues

Remember the biphasic dose response we discussed earlier—more isn't always better. There's a point of diminishing returns, after which additional exposure provides no added benefit and may potentially inhibit some of the positive effects.

Signs you might be undertreating

- No noticeable effects after 2–3 weeks of consistent use

- Temporary benefits that fade quickly after each session

- Minimal sensation during treatment (no gentle warming)

Signs you might be overtreating

- Increased fatigue after sessions

- Skin irritation or excessive redness

- Feeling overstimulated or having trouble sleeping (if used in evening)

- Plateauing or declining benefits after initial improvement

The good news is that red light therapy has a wide therapeutic window, so minor variations in duration are unlikely to cause problems. Start in the middle of the recommended range and adjust based on your response.

Frequency: How Often to Treat?

How often should you use your red light therapy device? Research and clinical experience suggest these general guidelines:

Daily use (7 days/week)

- Best for: Skin rejuvenation, hair growth, mood enhancement, general wellness

- Benefits: Builds cumulative effects more quickly, establishes consistent routine

- Considerations: Requires more time commitment, may need reduced session duration

Every other day (3–4 days/week)

- Best for: Recovery from exercise, pain management, wound healing, energy enhancement

- Benefits: Allows cellular regenerative processes to complete between sessions

- Considerations: Good balance for most applications, more sustainable long-term

Targeted intensive use (2x daily for specific conditions)

- Best for: Acute injuries, significant pain flares, accelerated healing needs

- Benefits: Can speed initial improvement for urgent situations

- Considerations: Should typically be reduced to standard frequency after initial intensive period (1–2 weeks)

Many users find that daily use during the initial 1–2 months helps establish the habit and build momentum with visible results, after which they may transition to a maintenance schedule of 3–5 times per week.

For specific conditions, optimal frequency can vary:

- **Pain and inflammation:** Start with daily sessions during acute phases, then 3–4 times weekly for maintenance

- **Skin rejuvenation:** 5–7 times weekly for initial improvements, then 3–5 times weekly for maintenance

- **Hair growth:** 5–7 times weekly consistently (results require regular ongoing treatment)

- **Recovery from exercise:** 3–5 times weekly, ideally immediately after intense workouts

- **Sleep improvement:** 1–2 hours before bedtime, 4–7 times weekly

- **Energy enhancement:** Morning sessions, 3–5 times weekly

- **Cognitive function:** Morning or midday sessions, 3–7 times weekly

Coverage: Targeting the Right Areas

Where you apply red light therapy depends on your goals, but there are some important principles to consider:

Direct Application: For most conditions, direct application to the target area is the most effective method. Point the light directly at the area of concern (such as a skin issue, painful joint, or injured muscle).

Systemic Benefits: Some benefits, particularly energy enhancement, sleep improvement, and general wellness, can be achieved by treating large, blood-rich areas of the body, such as the torso, back, and legs. These areas have high blood flow, which can help distribute the benefits throughout the body.

Strategic Coverage for Whole-Body Benefits: If you are using a smaller device for general wellness, prioritize these high-value areas:

1. **Abdomen and lower back:** Rich in blood vessels and close to vital organs
2. **Upper back and chest:** Large muscles and proximity to heart and lungs
3. **Legs (front and back):** Large muscle groups with extensive blood flow
4. **Head and neck:** For cognitive benefits, circulation, and thyroid function

Stacking vs. Rotating Areas: You can either:

- **Stacking:** Treat all target areas during each session (best for smaller devices or specific issues)

- **Rotating:** Cycle through different body areas on different days (more time-efficient for whole-body benefits)

For most users, I recommend starting with direct application to your primary areas of concern, then expanding to more general coverage as you establish your routine.

Timing: When to Use Red Light Therapy

The time of day you use your device can significantly impact certain benefits:

Morning Sessions (6 a.m.–12 p.m.) are ideal for:

- Energy enhancement
- Metabolism support
- Focus and cognitive function
- Athletic performance (pre-workout)

Midday Sessions (12 p.m.–5 p.m.) work well for:

- General wellness
- Pain management

- Skin treatments
- Recovery from morning workouts

Evening Sessions (5 p.m.–10 p.m.) are best for:

- Sleep improvement (1–2 hours before bed)
- Relaxation and stress reduction
- Recovery from afternoon/evening workouts
- Joint pain relief before bed

Some users report that evening sessions too close to bedtime (within 30 minutes) can sometimes feel stimulating, so experiment to find what works for your body. For sleep benefits, treatments 1–2 hours before bed tend to work best.

Combining With Other Activities

Red light therapy can be strategically combined with other activities:

Before Exercise

- May enhance performance and endurance
- Can prepare muscles and joints for activity
- Consider 5–15-minute sessions before workouts

RED LIGHT THERAPY

After Exercise

- Accelerates recovery and reduces soreness
- Helps reduce inflammation from intense training
- Most effective within 1 hour post-workout

During Meditation or Breathwork

- The quiet time and gentle warmth complement mindfulness practices
- May enhance stress reduction benefits

With Stretching or Yoga

- The warmth can help improve flexibility
- Complements the recovery aspects of these practices

Before Bed Routine

- Pairs well with reading, journaling, or gentle stretching
- Helps signal the body to prepare for sleep
- Avoid screens during this time for maximum benefit

Specific Protocols for Common Goals

Now let's create specific protocols for the most common goals people have with red light therapy.

These protocols assume a midrange device with both red and near-infrared capabilities but can be adapted to your specific device.

Protocol #1: Pain Relief and Inflammation

Best for: Joint pain, muscle soreness, inflammatory conditions, injuries

Setup

- **Distance:** 6–8 inches from target area

- **Wavelengths:** Combined red (660 nm) and near-infrared (850 nm)

- **Duration:** 10–20 minutes per treatment area

- **Frequency:** Daily for acute issues; 3–5 times weekly for maintenance

- **Coverage:** Direct application to painful area plus surrounding tissue (3–4 inches beyond pain site)

- **Timing:** Any time of day works; consider before bed for pain that disrupts sleep

Special considerations

- For acute injuries (within 48 hours), combine with cold therapy first, then use red light

- For chronic joint issues, consistent long-term use yields best results

- For deep tissue pain (like back pain), longer sessions (15–20 minutes) with near-infrared wavelengths work best

Signs it's working

- Reduced pain intensity within 3–7 sessions

- Increased range of motion

- Decreased dependency on pain medications

- Reduced visible swelling or redness

- More consistent relief with ongoing use

Protocol #2: Skin Rejuvenation and Anti-Aging

Best for: Fine lines, wrinkles, skin tone/texture, sun damage, minor blemishes

Setup

- **Distance:** 6–12 inches from face/skin

- **Wavelengths:** Primary focus on red (630–660 nm) with some near-infrared (850 nm)

- **Duration:** 10–15 minutes per treatment area

- **Frequency:** 5–7 times weekly for first month; 3–5 times weekly for maintenance

- **Coverage:** Full face, neck, décolletage, or other target areas
- **Timing:** Any time of day is effective; morning or evening routines work well

Special considerations

- Remove makeup and skincare products before treatment for better light penetration
- Eyes can remain open but avoid staring directly at LEDs
- Results are cumulative and typically noticeable after 4–6 weeks of consistent use
- Combine with good skincare practices including sun protection

Signs it's working

- Initial "glow" effect after sessions (increased circulation)
- Gradually improved skin texture within 2–4 weeks
- Reduction in fine lines around eyes and mouth by 8–12 weeks
- More even skin tone and reduced redness
- Improved moisture retention and plumpness

Protocol #3: Energy Enhancement and Fatigue Reduction

Best for: Low energy, fatigue, seasonal mood changes, productivity support

Setup

- **Distance:** 6–12 inches

- **Wavelengths:** Emphasis on near-infrared (850 nm) with some red (660 nm)

- **Duration:** 10–15 minutes per treatment area

- **Frequency:** 3–5 times weekly

- **Coverage:** Torso (abdomen and upper back/chest) are priority areas

- **Timing:** Morning sessions (within 2 hours of waking) yield best results

Special considerations

- Consistency matters more than intensity for energy benefits

- Hydration enhances results (drink water before and after sessions)

- Can be combined with morning sunlight exposure for enhanced circadian benefits

- Avoid late evening sessions if using for energy (can be too stimulating)

Signs it's working

- More consistent energy levels throughout the day
- Reduced afternoon energy crashes
- Less dependency on caffeine or stimulants
- Improved mental clarity alongside physical energy
- More stable mood and motivation

Protocol #4: Sleep Improvement

Best for: Trouble falling asleep, sleep quality issues, circadian rhythm support

Setup

- **Distance:** 12–18 inches
- **Wavelengths:** Balanced red (660 nm) and near-infrared (850 nm)
- **Duration:** 10–15 minutes
- **Frequency:** 4–7 times weekly
- **Coverage:** Full-body exposure is ideal; prioritize abdomen, chest, and head if using smaller device
- **Timing:** 1–2 hours before bedtime is optimal

Special considerations

- Combine with good sleep hygiene practices.
- Dimming other lights during and after treatment enhances effects.
- Avoid screen use during and after red light therapy session.
- Consider pairing with relaxation techniques (deep breathing, gentle stretching).

Signs it's working

- Reduced time to fall asleep
- Fewer nighttime awakenings
- More refreshed feeling upon waking
- More consistent sleep schedule
- Improved dream recall (indicates better REM sleep)

Protocol #5: Athletic Recovery and Performance

Best for: Workout recovery, reduced soreness, improved training capacity, injury prevention

Setup

- **Distance:** 6–12 inches
- **Wavelengths:** Emphasis on near-infrared (850 nm) with some red (660 nm)

- **Duration:** 10–20 minutes per treatment area
- **Frequency:** 3–5 times weekly, ideally after workouts
- **Coverage:** Target primary muscle groups used in training; rotate through different areas
- **Timing:** Within 1 hour post-workout for recovery; morning of competition for performance

Special considerations

- For recovery, use immediately after training when possible
- For performance, use 3–6 hours before competition
- Hydration enhances circulation benefits
- Can be combined with other recovery modalities (compression, light stretching)

Signs it's working

- Reduced delayed onset muscle soreness (DOMS)
- Faster return to training readiness
- Improved workout consistency

- Enhanced endurance or strength in subsequent workouts
- Better muscle pump and vascularity

Adapting Protocols to Your Device

Not all devices are created equal, so you'll need to adapt these protocols based on your specific device's capabilities:

For lower-power devices (under 30 mW/cm²):

- Increase treatment time by 25–50%
- Decrease treatment distance if possible
- Prioritize consistency over intensity
- Focus on smaller treatment areas

For higher-power devices (over 60 mW/cm²):

- Treatment times can be reduced by 25–30%
- Consider slightly increased treatment distance
- Monitor for signs of overtreatment
- Take advantage of ability to treat larger areas effectively

For single-wavelength devices

- If red-only (630–660 nm): Emphasize skin, surface circulation, and superficial pain

- If NIR-only (810–850 nm): Focus on deeper tissue, joints, muscles, and cognitive applications

For smaller treatment area devices

- Prioritize direct application to primary concern areas

- Consider multiple shorter sessions to cover different areas

- Rotate through body areas on different days

Tracking Your Results: The Measurement Framework

How do you know if your protocol is working? Establish baseline measurements before starting, then track progress regularly:

For pain and inflammation

- Rate pain on 0–10 scale daily

- Track range of motion with simple measurements

- Note medication usage and changes

- Take photos of visible inflammation or redness

For skin health

- Take well-lit before photos (same lighting/angle/time of day)
- Track specific concerns (wrinkles, spots, texture) on 0–10 scale
- Note changes in skincare routine or product needs
- Document compliments or observations from others

For energy and performance

- Rate energy levels throughout day (morning/afternoon/evening)
- Track workout performance and recovery time
- Note sleep quality correlation
- Measure caffeine or stimulant dependency

For sleep

- Record time to fall asleep
- Track nighttime awakenings
- Rate morning refreshment on 0–10 scale
- Use sleep tracking device if available

Use the self-assessment you completed in Chapter 1 as your baseline, and revisit it every 30 days to measure progress.

Conclusion

The protocols outlined in this chapter provide evidence-based starting points, but the most effective approach will always be personalized to your specific needs, goals, and response.

Begin with the protocol most aligned with your primary goal, follow it consistently for at least 30 days, and track your results. From there, you can refine based on your experience—adjusting duration, frequency, coverage, and timing to optimize your results.

Remember that many benefits of red light therapy are cumulative and develop over time. While some effects (like temporary pain relief or skin glow) may be noticeable immediately, the most significant improvements typically emerge after 4–12 weeks of consistent use.

In the next chapter, we'll dive into our 30-day kickstart plan—a comprehensive day-by-day guide to establishing your red light therapy practice and maximizing your results from the very beginning.

Chapter 6: The 30-Day Kickstart Plan– Day by Day Guide

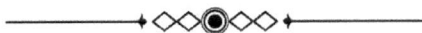

When I first started using red light therapy, I felt as though I was wandering in the dark (ironically enough). I had this powerful tool but no clear roadmap for how to use it effectively. I would change my approach every few days, jumping between different protocols I had read about online, never giving any single approach enough time to work. The result? Mediocre benefits and a nagging feeling that I was missing out on the full potential of this technology.

This pattern is incredibly common. People invest in quality devices but then flounder with inconsistent or suboptimal usage patterns. It's like buying a Ferrari but never learning how to drive stick—you might still get around, but you're missing the real experience.

That's why I have created this 30-day kickstart plan. It is designed to take the guesswork out of starting your red light therapy journey, providing a clear, structured approach that builds momentum while teaching you to listen to your body's responses.

This isn't just a rigid protocol; it's a learning experience that will help you discover how red light therapy works best for your unique body and goals. By the end of these 30 days, you will have established a sustainable practice and gained the knowledge to fine-tune your approach for maximum benefit.

Before You Begin: Preparation for Success

Before diving into Day 1, take some time to set yourself up for success:

1. Establish Your Baseline

Remember the self-assessment from Chapter 1? If you haven't completed it yet, do so now. Rate yourself from 1 to 1–10 in these key areas:

- Energy level throughout the day
- Sleep quality
- Recovery time after physical activity
- Pain levels (note specific problem areas)
- Skin health and appearance
- Mental clarity and focus

- Overall sense of vitality

Take "before" photos of any visible conditions you're hoping to improve (skin concerns, hair thinning, etc.). Use consistent lighting and angles so you can make accurate comparisons later.

2. Set Up Your Space

Create a dedicated area for your red light therapy sessions:

- Choose a comfortable location with enough space to move around
- Ensure access to a timer or clock
- Consider a mirror for proper positioning if treating specific areas
- Have a comfortable chair or mat if you'll be sitting or lying down
- Keep water nearby (hydration enhances results)

3. Schedule Your Sessions

Decide when you will do your red light therapy sessions and block that time on your calendar. Morning sessions tend to work well for energy and metabolism, while evening sessions (1–2 hours before bed) can support sleep. Whatever time you choose, consistency matters more than perfect timing.

4. Set Realistic Expectations

Remember that while some effects (such as pain relief or skin glow) may be noticeable within days, the most significant benefits typically emerge after 4 to 12 weeks of consistent use. This 30-day plan is just the beginning of your journey.

Week 1: Establishing the Foundation (Days 1–7)

The first week focuses on building the habit, finding your comfort zone with the device, and establishing your baseline response.

Day 1: First Contact

Today's Focus: Familiarizing yourself with your device and establishing comfort.

Morning

- Unpack and set up your device according to manufacturer instructions
- Read safety guidelines carefully
- Test the device briefly to ensure proper function

Session Plan

- Start with a short 5-minute session at the recommended distance.

- Focus on a single area (the abdomen or upper back are good starting points).

- Notice the sensation, warmth, and any immediate effects.

- Note your experience in your journal.

Evening reflection

- How did your body feel during and after the session?

- Any immediate effects (relaxation, warmth, energy shift)?

- What questions or concerns arose from this first experience?

Day 2: Expanding Exposure

Today's Focus: Increasing duration and adding a second treatment area.

Session Plan

Increase to 8 minutes per treatment area.

Treat two areas: repeat yesterday's area plus add one new area.

Maintain consistent distance from device.

Focus on your breathing and relaxation during treatment.

Journal prompts

How does today's longer session compare to yesterday?

Any differences in how your body responds to different treatment areas?

How does your energy feel a few hours after treatment?

Day 3: Finding Your Rhythm

Today's Focus: Establishing a consistent time for your sessions.

Session Plan

10 minutes per treatment area.

Treat the same two areas as yesterday.

Schedule your session at the time you plan to maintain throughout the program.

Begin conscious relaxation during your session.

Journal prompts

How does the timing of your session affect your experience?

Are you noticing any patterns in how you feel during or after treatment?

Is the current session time practical for your daily routine?

Day 4: Rest and Reflection

Today's Focus: Learning the importance of off days and observation.

Session Plan

No red light therapy today.

Instead, spend 10 minutes reviewing your notes from the first three days.

Notice how your body feels without treatment today.

Journal prompts

Do you notice any lingering effects from previous sessions?

How is your sleep, energy, or specific condition today compared to before starting?

What questions do you have after your first few experiences?

Day 5: Introducing Targeted Application

Today's Focus: Applying red light to your primary area of concern.

Session Plan

10 minutes on general areas (as in Days 2–3)

Add 10 minutes focused specifically on your primary concern area:

For skin: face and neck

For pain: the specific painful area

For energy: abdomen and chest

For sleep: upper back and chest

For hair growth: scalp

Pay attention to any differences in sensation or response

Journal prompts

How does your target area respond compared to general application?

Any immediate effects specific to your main concern?

Is the current session duration comfortable or challenging to maintain?

Day 6: Optimizing Position and Distance

Today's Focus: Experimenting with treatment distance.

Session Plan

Maintain 10 minutes per treatment area

First area: Try positioning slightly closer than previous days

Second area: Try positioning slightly farther than previous days

Note differences in sensation and comfort

Journal prompts

How does changing distance affect warmth, comfort, and overall experience?

Which distance feels most effective for different body areas?

How is your consistency with daily sessions so far?

Day 7: Full Assessment and Week 1 Review

Today's Focus: Evaluating your first week and planning adjustments.

Session Plan

- 10 minutes per treatment area

- Use your preferred distance based on Day 6 experiments
- Treat all primary areas of concern

Evening Review

- Complete a full self-assessment (same format as your baseline)
- Compare to your starting point—note any changes, even subtle ones
- Review your journal entries from the week
- Identify any patterns in your response
- Plan any adjustments needed for Week 2

Week 2: Optimizing Your Approach (Days 8–14)

In Week 2, we'll refine your protocol based on your Week 1 experiences, increasing intensity while paying closer attention to your body's responses.

Day 8: Intensity Progression

Today's Focus: Safely increasing treatment intensity.

Session Plan

- Increase to 12–15 minutes per treatment area

- Slightly decrease distance if comfortable (based on Week 1 observations)
- Focus on your primary concern areas first, then general wellness areas
- Pay attention to any intensified responses

Journal prompts

- How does your body respond to increased intensity?
- Any new sensations or effects?
- Is the longer duration sustainable for your schedule?

Day 9: Wavelength Exploration

Today's Focus: Understanding different wavelength effects (if your device offers multiple wavelengths).

Session Plan

- For devices with separate red and near-infrared settings:
  - First 5 minutes: Red wavelengths only
  - Second 5 minutes: Near-infrared only
  - Final 5 minutes: Combined wavelengths
- If your device has only one wavelength, maintain your Day 8 protocol

- Note any differences in sensation or effect

Journal prompts

- Can you feel differences between wavelength settings?
- Which setting seems most effective for your specific goals?
- Any preferences emerging for different treatment areas?

Day 10: Time of Day Experiment

Today's Focus: Exploring how timing affects your results.

Session Plan

- Split your session into two shorter sessions (7–8 minutes each)
- First session: Morning or early afternoon
- Second session: Evening (at least 1–2 hours before bed)
- Use the same treatment areas and distance for both sessions

Journal prompts

- How do morning vs. evening sessions differ in feeling and effect?

- Which timing seems to better support your main goals?
- Do you notice any impact on energy, focus, or sleep from different timing?

Day 11: Synergy With Movement

Today's Focus: Combining red light therapy with gentle movement.

Session Plan

- 15 minutes total treatment time
- Incorporate gentle stretching, tai chi movements, or simple yoga poses during your session
- Focus red light on areas you're actively moving or stretching
- Maintain deep, mindful breathing throughout

Journal prompts

- How does movement enhance or change your experience?
- Any increased warmth, circulation, or flexibility when combining movement?
- Would this combination fit well into your regular routine?

Day 12: Recovery Focus

Today's Focus: Using red light therapy specifically for recovery.

Session Plan

- Schedule session after physical activity (workout, walking, gardening, etc.)
- Focus 15 minutes on the muscle groups most used in your activity
- Compare recovery sensation to your usual post-activity feeling

Journal prompts

- How does your post-activity recovery compare to normal?
- Any reduction in expected soreness or fatigue?
- How quickly do you feel ready for more activity?

Day 13: Mindfulness Integration

Today's Focus: Enhancing results through focused awareness.

Session Plan

- 15 minutes on primary treatment areas

- Practice deep breathing and body scanning during treatment
- Consciously direct attention to the area being treated
- Imagine light penetrating deeply and energizing cells

Journal prompts

- How does mental focus affect your experience?
- Any difference in warmth or sensation with focused attention?
- Does the mindfulness aspect make the session more or less enjoyable?

Day 14: Week 2 Assessment and Progress Check

Today's Focus: Measuring progress and refining your approach.

Session Plan

- Full-protocol session (15 minutes per key area)
- Use your current preferred settings and approach
- Take progress photos for visual comparison

Evening Review

- Complete full self-assessment
- Compare to baseline and Week 1 review
- Note improvements or changes, even subtle ones
- Review journal entries for patterns and insights

Week 3: Integration and Expansion (Days 15–21)

In Week 3, we'll integrate red light therapy more fully into your lifestyle and explore complementary practices to enhance results.

Day 15–21: Enhancing Your Practice

Over this week, you'll explore several enhancements to your basic protocol:

- **Hydration Enhancement:** Drink plenty of water before and after sessions to maximize benefits
- **Circulation Boosting:** Add brief warm-up movements before treatment
- **Targeted Intensive Treatment:** Focus longer sessions on your primary concern

- **Relaxation Enhancement:** Combine evening sessions with stress-reduction techniques

- **Nutrition Synergy:** Support your practice with anti-inflammatory foods

- **Intuitive Application:** Learn to listen to your body's needs and adjust treatment accordingly

Each day, maintain your core protocol while adding one enhancement. By Week 3's end, complete another full assessment to measure your progress.

Week 4: Fine-Tuning for Maximum Results (Days 22–30)

In the final week, you'll refine your personal protocol based on everything you've learned, ensuring that you have a sustainable practice to continue beyond the 30-day kickstart.

Days 22–29: Personalization and Optimization

During this week, focus on:

- **Personalized Protocol Design:** Create your ideal routine based on your experiences.

- **Morning Energizer:** Optimize morning use for energy and metabolism.

- **Performance Enhancement:** Time sessions to support physical activities.

- **Deep Recovery:** Maximize recovery benefits after exertion.

- **Sleep Optimization:** Fine-tune evening sessions for better sleep.

- **Skin and Aesthetics Focus:** Refine your approach for visible improvements.

- **Stress and Balance:** Use red light therapy for mental well-being.

By the end of Week 4, you'll have a comprehensive understanding of how red light therapy works best for your unique needs.

Day 30: Celebration and Future Planning

Today's Focus: Assessing your 30-day journey and planning for continued success.

Session Plan

- Complete your personal favorite protocol
- Take final progress photos
- Implement any final refinements

Final Assessment

- Complete detailed self-assessment in all areas
- Compare to baseline and weekly reviews
- Create side-by-side photo comparisons
- Review entire journal for patterns and insights

Reflection and Planning

- What were your most significant improvements?
- Which aspects of red light therapy were most valuable for you?
- What surprised you most about this experience?
- How will you continue your practice beyond the 30 days?
- What long-term goals will you set for the next 60-90 days?

Extending Beyond 30 Days: Your Sustainable Practice

Congratulations on completing the 30-day kickstart! By now, you should have a clear understanding of how red light therapy works for your unique body and goals. You have developed a personalized protocol and established a consistent practice.

Most people find these maintenance schedules effective after the initial 30-day intensive program:

For general wellness and prevention

- 3–4 sessions per week
- 10–15 minutes per session
- Focus on rotating different body areas

For specific conditions or concerns

- 4–5 sessions per week
- 15–20 minutes per session
- Primary focus on target areas with some general application

When you encounter new health challenges or goals, you can always return to more intensive protocols temporarily. Trust the body awareness you've developed during the 30-day program to guide your ongoing practice.

In the next chapter, we will explore advanced strategies to take your practice even further, including the combination of red light therapy with other modalities for enhanced results.

Chapter 7:
Beyond the Basics–Advanced Strategies for Optimal Results

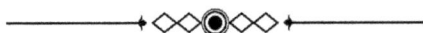

By now, you've established a solid foundation for your red light therapy practice. You understand the fundamentals of how it works, have selected an appropriate device, and implemented a consistent protocol through the 30-day kickstart plan. You may already be experiencing noticeable benefits.

But what if you could take these results even further?

That's what this chapter is all about—advanced strategies that can amplify your results and help you break through plateaus. These approaches go beyond basic device usage to create synergistic effects through strategic combinations with other health modalities, timing optimizations, and protocol refinements.

I should note that while the basic protocols in previous chapters are supported by substantial research, some of the advanced strategies we'll explore here are more experimental. They represent cutting-edge approaches being used by biohackers, progressive clinicians, and health optimizers—sometimes ahead of published research. I'll be clear about which strategies have strong scientific backing versus those based more on clinical experience and emerging evidence.

Synergistic Combinations: Red Light + Other Modalities

One of the most exciting aspects of red light therapy is how well it pairs with other health practices. These combinations often create effects that are greater than the sum of their parts.

Red Light Therapy + Cold Exposure

The combination of cold exposure (cold showers, ice baths, cryotherapy) followed by red light therapy has become a favorite among biohackers and athletes for good reason.

The Science: Cold exposure increases mitochondrial biogenesis (the creation of new mitochondria) through hormetic stress, while red light therapy improves mitochondrial function. Together, they may create a powerful one-two punch for cellular energy.

How to Implement

1. Begin with 1 to 5 minutes of cold exposure (cold shower, ice bath, or local ice application).
2. Follow immediately with 10 to 15 minutes of red light therapy.
3. Focus the red light on the same areas that received cold treatment.
4. Pay attention to the sensation of increased blood flow and warmth.

Who Benefits Most: Athletes, individuals with inflammation or pain issues, and anyone seeking enhanced energy and metabolic benefits.

Red Light Therapy + Heat (Sauna)

While seemingly opposite to the cold approach, combining red light therapy with sauna sessions can also create synergistic benefits.

The Science: Sauna therapy increases heat shock proteins, enhances detoxification pathways, and improves cardiovascular function. Red light therapy complements these effects through improved mitochondrial function and cellular energy production.

How to Implement

Option 1—Sauna First

1. 15–20 minute sauna session at 150–180°F
2. Cool down period (5–10 minutes)
3. 15-minute red light therapy session

Option 2—Red Light First

1. 10–15 minute red light therapy session
2. 15–20 minute sauna session
3. Cool down and hydration

Who Benefits Most: Those focusing on detoxification, skin health, stress reduction, and cardiovascular benefits.

Red Light Therapy + Exercise

Strategically combining red light therapy with your workout routine can enhance both performance and recovery.

The Science: Pre-workout red light therapy may increase nitric oxide production, enhancing blood flow to muscles and improving energy availability. Post-workout applications can accelerate recovery by reducing inflammation and oxidative stress while supporting mitochondrial energy production for repair processes.

How to Implement

Pre-workout protocol

1. 5–10 minutes of red light therapy on major muscle groups you'll be training
2. Begin workout within 30–60 minutes of treatment
3. Focus on proper warm-up to maintain increased blood flow

Post-workout protocol

1. Complete workout
2. Hydrate and consume protein if appropriate
3. 10–20 minutes of red light therapy on worked muscles within 1 hour
4. Focus on breathing and relaxation during treatment

Who Benefits Most: Athletes, fitness enthusiasts, and those using exercise therapeutically for health conditions.

Red Light Therapy + Fasting

The combination of red light therapy during fasting periods has gained popularity among those practicing intermittent or extended fasting.

The Science: Fasting triggers autophagy (cellular cleanup processes) and metabolic switching to fat metabolism. Red light therapy may support these processes by providing cellular energy through non-food pathways (direct photonic stimulation of mitochondria), potentially making fasting easier while enhancing its benefits.

How to Implement

For intermittent fasting (16:8, 18:6, etc.):

1. Morning session: 10–15 minutes during fasted state
2. Focus on abdomen, liver area, and muscles
3. Drink water before and after treatment

Who Benefits Most: Those practicing intermittent or extended fasting for metabolic health, weight management, or longevity benefits.

Red Light Therapy + Targeted Supplementation

Certain supplements may enhance the effects of red light therapy through complementary mechanisms.

The Science: Some compounds support the same cellular processes that red light therapy enhances, potentially creating synergistic effects. The most promising combinations include:

Mitochondrial Support Supplements

- **CoQ10/Ubiquinol**: A key component of the electron transport chain stimulated by red light

- **PQQ (Pyrroloquinoline quinone)**: Supports mitochondrial biogenesis

- **L-carnitine:** Enhances fatty acid transport into mitochondria

- **Creatine:** Supports cellular energy reserves and ATP production

How to Implement

1. Consider adding 1–2 targeted supplements based on your primary goals

2. Take most mitochondrial supplements 30–60 minutes before red light sessions

3. Maintain consistent supplementation for at least 30 days alongside red light therapy

4. Monitor for enhanced or accelerated benefits

Who Benefits Most: Those focusing on mitochondrial health, anti-aging, skin rejuvenation, or energy enhancement.

Advanced Timing Strategies

Beyond basic combinations with other modalities, the precise timing of your red light therapy can significantly impact results.

Circadian Optimization

Aligning red light therapy with your body's natural circadian rhythms may enhance specific benefits.

The Science: Different bodily systems are more responsive at different times of day. Morning light exposure helps set circadian rhythms, while evening red light (which doesn't suppress melatonin like blue light) may support transition to sleep. Additionally, your skin's ability to repair and regenerate peaks during early sleep phases.

How to Implement

Morning Protocol (within 30–60 minutes of waking)

1. 5–10 minutes of natural sunlight exposure if possible (sets primary circadian signals)
2. 10–15 minutes of red light therapy focusing on:
   o Face and eyes (do not stare directly at lights but allow ambient exposure with eyes open)

o Abdomen for metabolic activation
o Large muscle groups for energy
3. Stay well-hydrated and maintain consistent morning timing

Evening Protocol (1–2 hours before bed)

1. Reduce blue light exposure (screens, bright white lights) first
2. 10–15 minutes of red light therapy focusing on:
   o Full body for general recovery
   o Brain (transcranial application) for relaxation
   o Areas needing repair or regeneration
3. Follow with relaxing activities (reading, gentle stretching, meditation)

Who Benefits Most: Those with circadian disruption (shift workers, travelers), sleep issues, seasonal mood changes, or those seeking to optimize overall rhythms.

Pulsed Protocols

Instead of continuous daily application, some advanced users implement pulsed protocols—intensive use for several days followed by rest periods.

The Science: Hormetic stressors (beneficial stressors that trigger positive adaptations) often work best with recovery periods. Pulsed protocols may prevent habituation (decreased response over time) and potentially enhance long-term results.

How to Implement

5–2 Protocol

1. 5 days of intensive treatment (daily, potentially multiple sessions)
2. 2 days complete rest from red light therapy
3. Repeat cycle

Intensity Cycling

1. Week 1–2: Daily sessions (10–15 minutes)
2. Week 3: Increased intensity (15–20 minutes, slightly closer distance)
3. Week 4: Reduced frequency (3–4 times weekly) but maintained intensity
4. Repeat cycle

Who Benefits Most: Those who've reached plateaus with standard protocols, performance-focused individuals, and those addressing specific acute conditions.

Tissue-Specific Advanced Strategies

Different tissues respond optimally to slightly different protocols. Here are advanced strategies for specific targets:

Deep Tissue Optimization

For reaching deeper tissues like large joints, visceral organs, and deeper muscles:

The Science: Near-infrared wavelengths (810–850 nm) penetrate more deeply than red (630-660 nm). Additionally, pressure techniques can temporarily displace surface blood and water, allowing light to penetrate more effectively to deeper structures.

How to Implement

1. Use primarily near-infrared wavelengths
2. Apply gentle pressure to compress surface tissues when appropriate
3. Increase session duration by 25–50% for deep targets
4. Consider multiple angles to reach the same deep structure
5. Stay well-hydrated to optimize tissue light transmission

Application Example: Deep Knee Joint

1. Near-infrared wavelengths at 6–8 inches

2. 10 minutes from front of knee
3. 10 minutes from back of knee
4. 5 minutes from each side
5. Gentle movement during latter portion of treatment

Who Benefits Most: Those with deep joint pain, internal organ concerns, or deep muscle injuries.

Brain Optimization (Transcranial Application)

For cognitive function, mood, and neurological support:

The Science: Near-infrared light can penetrate the skull and reach brain tissue, potentially supporting mitochondrial function in neurons, reducing neuroinflammation, and increasing brain-derived neurotrophic factor (BDNF).

How to Implement

1. Use near-infrared wavelengths (810–850 nm) exclusively
2. Position light 1–6 inches from skull
3. Target specific regions based on goals:
   o Forehead/prefrontal cortex: Executive function, mood, decision-making
   o Temporal regions: Memory, language processing

o Top of head: Motor coordination, overall brain energy

4. 10–15 minutes per region, potentially rotating regions on different days

5. Stay well-hydrated and consider combining with cognitive tasks during treatment

Who Benefits Most: Those focusing on cognitive performance, mood support, age-related cognitive changes, or recovery from brain injuries.

Skin Rejuvenation Advanced Protocols

For enhanced aesthetic results and dermal remodeling:

The Science: Alternating wavelengths, distances, and combining with specific topicals may enhance skin regeneration and collagen production. Certain topical ingredients become more effective when used before or after red light therapy.

How to Implement

Pre-treatment preparation

1. Gentle exfoliation to remove dead skin cells

2. Thorough cleansing with non-blocking cleanser

3. Optional: Hyaluronic acid serum application (enhances hydration)

Multi-angle protocol

1. 5 minutes at 12 inches (broader, more diffuse coverage)
2. 5 minutes at 6 inches (more intense, targeted exposure)
3. Final 5 minutes at 12 inches

Wavelength cycling protocol

1. 5 minutes red wavelengths (630–660 nm) for surface issues
2. 5 minutes near-infrared (810–850 nm) for deeper dermal layers
3. 5 minutes combined wavelengths

Who Benefits Most: Those focusing on anti-aging, skin texture, tone concerns, scarring, or specific dermatological conditions.

Seasonal Strategies and Adaptations

Just as our ancestors adapted to seasonal light changes, we can optimize red light therapy seasonally:

Winter Optimization

During darker months with less natural sunlight:

1. **Increased frequency:** Daily sessions to compensate for reduced natural light

2. **Morning emphasis:** Early day sessions to support circadian rhythms

3. **Extended duration:** 25–50% longer sessions for immune and mood support

4. **Full-spectrum approach:** Combine with broad-spectrum light therapy for mood (separate from red light therapy)

Summer Adaptations

During months with abundant natural light:

1. **Strategic timing:** Early morning or evening sessions to complement natural light

2. **Targeted application:** Focus on specific concerns rather than general light exposure

3. **Recovery emphasis:** Focus on post-sun-exposure recovery and repair

4. **Skin support:** Enhanced protocols for UV-exposed areas

Breaking Through Plateaus

Even the most effective protocols can reach plateaus. Here are advanced strategies for continuing progress:

Protocol Cycling

Implementation

1. 3 weeks on your standard protocol
2. 1 week of "protocol shock"—significantly different approach:
   o Different timing
   o Different distance/intensity
   o Focus on previously secondary areas
   o Combine with different complementary practices
3. Return to standard or hybrid protocol

Hormetic Stress Addition

Implementation

1. Add new hormetic stress alongside red light therapy:
   o Brief intense exercise bursts
   o Hot/cold contrast
   o Breathwork (hypoxic training)
   o New movement patterns
2. Start with brief exposures and monitor adaptive response
3. Gradually increase intensity of added stressor

Device Stacking

For those with multiple devices or access to different types:

Implementation

1. Layer different devices for targeted areas:
   - o Targeted device for specific concern
   - o Panel for broader coverage
   - o Consider different wavelengths with different devices

2. Experiment with simultaneous versus sequential use

3. Create priority rotation if using multiple targeted devices

Tracking Advanced Protocols

As you implement more complex strategies, tracking becomes even more important:

Biomarker Monitoring

Consider tracking relevant biomarkers based on your goals:

- HRV (heart rate variability) for stress and recovery
- Sleep metrics via tracking devices

- Blood markers when appropriate and available
- Hormone panels for hormone-related applications

Advanced Journaling Framework

Implementation

1. Pre-session metrics
   - Energy rating (1–10)
   - Stress level (1–10)
   - Target concern rating
   - Sleep quality previous night
   - Other relevant activities that day
2. Session details
   - Protocol used (including all variables)
   - Complementary practices
   - Subjective experience notes
   - Unusual sensations or responses
3. Post-session metrics
   - Immediate effects (0–6 hours)
   - Next-day effects
   - Cumulative weekly observations
   - Photos for visible concerns

Conclusion: The Experimental Mindset

As you explore these advanced strategies, maintain what I call the "experimental mindset"—curious, methodical, and attentive to results without attachment to expectations. Track what works for your unique body, be willing to adjust based on results, and remember that sometimes simpler protocols deliver better outcomes than more complex approaches.

These advanced strategies represent the cutting edge of red light therapy practice, combining research, clinical experience, and pioneering self-experimentation from the biohacking community. Some will eventually be validated by formal research, while others may be refined or replaced as our understanding evolves.

The beauty of red light therapy is that it offers a remarkably safe space for such exploration and personalization. Unlike many interventions with narrow therapeutic windows and significant risks, red light therapy's safety profile allows for creative protocol development with minimal downside risk.

In the next chapter, we will explore real-world success stories—case studies of individuals who have experienced remarkable results with red light therapy for various conditions. These stories will illustrate how the principles and protocols we have covered translate into meaningful health improvements for real people.

How to Implement

Option 1—Sauna First

1. 15–20 minute sauna session at 150–180°F
2. Cool down period (5–10 minutes)
3. 15-minute red light therapy session

Option 2—Red Light First

1. 10–15 minute red light therapy session
2. 15–20 minute sauna session
3. Cool down and hydration

Who Benefits Most: Those focusing on detoxification, skin health, stress reduction, and cardiovascular benefits.

Red Light Therapy + Exercise

Strategically combining red light therapy with your workout routine can enhance both performance and recovery.

The Science: Pre-workout red light therapy may increase nitric oxide production, enhancing blood flow to muscles and improving energy availability. Post-workout applications can accelerate recovery by reducing inflammation and oxidative stress while supporting mitochondrial energy production for repair processes.

How to Implement

Pre-workout protocol

1. 5–10 minutes of red light therapy on major muscle groups you'll be training
2. Begin workout within 30–60 minutes of treatment
3. Focus on proper warm-up to maintain increased blood flow

Post-workout protocol

1. Complete workout
2. Hydrate and consume protein if appropriate
3. 10–20 minutes of red light therapy on worked muscles within 1 hour
4. Focus on breathing and relaxation during treatment

Who Benefits Most: Athletes, fitness enthusiasts, and those using exercise therapeutically for health conditions.

Red Light Therapy + Fasting

The combination of red light therapy during fasting periods has gained popularity among those practicing intermittent or extended fasting.

The Science: Fasting triggers autophagy (cellular cleanup processes) and metabolic switching to fat metabolism. Red light therapy may support these processes by providing cellular energy through non-food pathways (direct photonic stimulation of mitochondria), potentially making fasting easier while enhancing its benefits.

How to Implement

For intermittent fasting (16:8, 18:6, etc.)

1. Morning session: 10–15 minutes during fasted state
2. Focus on abdomen, liver area, and muscles
3. Drink water before and after treatment

Who Benefits Most: Those practicing intermittent or extended fasting for metabolic health, weight management, or longevity benefits.

Red Light Therapy + Targeted Supplementation

Certain supplements may enhance the effects of red light therapy through complementary mechanisms.

The Science: Some compounds support the same cellular processes that red light therapy enhances, potentially creating synergistic effects. The most promising combinations include:

Mitochondrial Support Supplements

- **CoQ10/Ubiquinol:** A key component of the electron transport chain stimulated by red light

- **PQQ (Pyrroloquinoline quinone):** Supports mitochondrial biogenesis

- **L-carnitine:** Enhances fatty acid transport into mitochondria

- **Creatine:** Supports cellular energy reserves and ATP production

How to Implement

1. Consider adding 1–2 targeted supplements based on your primary goals

2. Take most mitochondrial supplements 30–60 minutes before red light sessions

3. Maintain consistent supplementation for at least 30 days alongside red light therapy

4. Monitor for enhanced or accelerated benefits

Who Benefits Most: Those focusing on mitochondrial health, anti-aging, skin rejuvenation, or energy enhancement.

Advanced Timing Strategies

Beyond basic combinations with other modalities, the precise timing of your red light therapy can significantly impact results.

Circadian Optimization

Aligning red light therapy with your body's natural circadian rhythms may enhance specific benefits.

The Science: Different bodily systems are more responsive at different times of day. Morning light exposure helps set circadian rhythms, while evening red light (which doesn't suppress melatonin like blue light) may support transition to sleep. Additionally, your skin's ability to repair and regenerate peaks during early sleep phases.

Chapter 8: Real Results—Success Stories and Case Studies

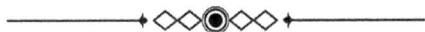

Throughout this book, we have explored the science behind red light therapy, practical protocols, and advanced strategies. However, there is something uniquely powerful about seeing how these principles translate into real-life transformations for actual people.

In this chapter, I will share authentic case studies from individuals who have experienced significant benefits from consistent use of red light therapy. These stories illustrate not only the potential outcomes but also the journey—including the challenges faced, adjustments made, and lessons learned along the way.

I have deliberately selected a diverse range of experiences across different ages, conditions, and goals to demonstrate the versatility of red light therapy. While each person's journey is unique, these stories reveal common patterns that can help guide your own practice.

For privacy reasons, some names have been changed, but all case studies are based on real experiences documented through interviews, photos, journals, and, in some cases, clinical measurements.

Athletic Performance and Recovery: Michael's Story

Background: Michael, 42, is a former college athlete who now works as an executive. He trains intensely 5 to 6 days a week, focusing on strength training and high-intensity interval cardio. He has been struggling with persistent muscle soreness, declining recovery capacity, and nagging joint issues that have affected both his performance and quality of life.

Initial Challenges: "In my 20s and early 30s, I could train hard, recover quickly, and feel great. By the time I turned 40, I was constantly sore, sleeping poorly, and felt as though my body was fighting against me. I was considering scaling back my training significantly, which was depressing because it is such an important part of my life and identity."

Red Light Protocol: Michael invested in a medium-sized panel device that emits both red and near-infrared wavelengths. His initial protocol:

- 15 minutes post-workout, focusing on trained muscle groups

- Distance: 12 inches

- Frequency: 4–5 times weekly following training sessions

- Combined with improved hydration and magnesium supplementation

Evolution and Adjustments: After three weeks with moderate results, Michael made these pivotal changes:

1. Added pre-workout sessions (10 minutes) focused on joints and chronically tight areas.

2. Increased post-workout sessions to 20 minutes.

3. Added specific focus on lower back and knees (previous injury sites).

4. Incorporated gentle movement during some sessions.

Six-Month Results

- Recovery time decreased from 48–72 hours to 24–36 hours for intense sessions.

- Morning stiffness reduced by approximately 70%.

- Sleep quality improved significantly (verified by wearable sleep tracker).

- Training volume increased by 15% without increased soreness.

- Chronic knee pain reduced from 6/10 to 2/10 on pain scale.

Key Insights From Michael: "The biggest surprise was how the benefits compound over time. The first month was good but not revolutionary. By month three, the differences were dramatic. Now at six months, I'm training harder at 42 than I was at 39, with better recovery. The key for me was consistency and the dual approach—using it both before and after workouts."

Chronic Pain Management: Sarah's Story

Background: Sarah, 58, elementary school teacher with a 15-year history of rheumatoid arthritis. Despite medication management, she experienced persistent pain and stiffness, particularly in her hands, wrists, and knees. This was affecting her quality of life and making classroom activities increasingly difficult.

Initial Challenges: "The hardest part was the unpredictability. Some mornings I couldn't button my shirt or open jars. As a teacher, I need my hands for everything from writing on the board to helping children with projects. I was taking pain medication daily just to function and still had to modify many activities."

Red Light Protocol: Sarah began with a modest handheld device, focusing on her hands and wrists, later adding a small panel for larger joints.

Initial protocol

- 10 minutes on each hand/wrist, morning and evening
- 10 minutes on each knee in the evening
- Distance: 6 inches
- Frequency: Daily for hands, 5 times weekly for knees
- Used primarily red wavelengths (660 nm) with some near-infrared

Evolution and Adjustments

1. Added gentle finger movements during hand treatments
2. Incorporated warm paraffin wax treatment before morning sessions

3. Extended knee sessions to 15 minutes with greater focus on near-infrared
4. Added weekend intensive sessions (20 minutes per area)

One-Year Results

- Morning stiffness duration decreased from 3+ hours to under 30 minutes

- Handgrip strength increased by 40% (measured with grip dynamometer)

- Pain medication usage reduced by approximately 60%

- Flare frequency decreased from bi-monthly to quarterly

- Range of motion in fingers increased significantly

Key Insights from Sarah: "Consistency was absolutely critical—I noticed that if I missed even two days, my symptoms would begin to return. The morning sessions made the biggest difference for my daily function, while the evening sessions seemed to help more with overnight pain and sleep quality."

Skin Transformation: Emma's Story

Background: Emma, 36, is a marketing executive with increasing concerns about premature aging, including fine lines, uneven skin tone, and post-inflammatory hyperpigmentation from adult acne. She had tried numerous skincare regimens with limited results and was considering more invasive procedures.

Initial Challenges: "I was frustrated with spending hundreds on serums and treatments that made big promises but delivered minimal results. My skin looked tired, and I had developed fine lines around my eyes that made me look perpetually exhausted. The acne scarring on my cheeks was particularly stubborn and affected my confidence in professional settings."

Red Light Protocol: Emma invested in a high-quality facial mask device that utilizes both red (630 nm) and near-infrared (830 nm) wavelengths:

Initial protocol:

- 20-minute daily sessions
- Combined wavelength setting
- Evening application after thorough cleansing

- Followed by simple, non-blocking moisturizer
- Consistent sunscreen use during the day

Evolution and Adjustments

1. Added gentle chemical exfoliation 2x weekly (not on the same day as red light).
2. Incorporated hyaluronic acid serum before treatment.
3. Added targeted handheld treatment for 5 extra minutes on hyperpigmentation areas.
4. Developed a weekly intensive protocol: gentle exfoliation, a 30-minute session, followed by peptide serum.

Six-Month Results

- Fine lines around eyes reduced by approximately 50–60%.
- Skin tone evenness significantly improved (documented in progress photos).
- Post-inflammatory hyperpigmentation lightened by 70–80%.
- Skin texture refinement is noticeable within the first 30 days.
- Two unexpected breakouts healed in half the usual time.

Key Insights from Emma: "The results were gradual but unmistakable. Around week three, people started commenting that I looked 'rested' or asked if I'd changed my makeup. By month three, I was using less foundation and concealer. The biggest surprise was how it helped new breakouts heal—what would normally be a two-week ordeal would resolve in days with targeted treatment."

Energy and Mood Enhancement: David's Story

Background: David, 45, a software engineer and father of three, struggled with seasonal energy fluctuations, afternoon crashes, and low mood during winter months. These issues were affecting both his work performance and family life, particularly during November through February.

Initial Challenges: "Winter was always rough. By 2 p.m., I'd hit a wall—mentally foggy, physically drained, and irritable. I was relying on constant caffeine, which affected my sleep, creating a vicious cycle. I tried everything from vitamin D supplements to light boxes with moderate benefits but still struggled through the darker months."

Red Light Protocol: David purchased a large panel device with both red and near-infrared capabilities:

Initial protocol

- 15-minute morning sessions (7:00–7:30 a.m.)
- Full-body exposure at 12–18 inches
- Emphasis on torso and head
- Combined wavelengths
- 5 times weekly (weekdays)

Evolution and Adjustments

1. Added brief midday "rescue" sessions (5 minutes) when afternoon crashes were imminent
2. Incorporated gentle movement during morning sessions
3. Added weekend evening sessions with focus on relaxation and sleep quality
4. Developed seasonal adjustments: longer sessions and higher frequency during winter months

Four-Month Results (including transition from fall to winter):

- Afternoon energy crashes reduced from daily to 1–2 times weekly

- Mood stability significantly improved (tracked in daily journal)

- Sleep onset time improved by average of 45 minutes

- Morning waking became easier and more consistent

- Caffeine consumption reduced by 50%

Key Insights from David: "The morning sessions were absolutely transformative—it was like creating an artificial sunrise for my body during those dark winter mornings. I noticed that timing was crucial; if I delayed my session until after 9 a.m., the benefits weren't as pronounced. The combination of movement during treatment seemed to amplify the energizing effects."

Sleep Quality Enhancement: Jennifer's Story

Background: Jennifer, 49, healthcare administrator with chronic sleep difficulties including trouble falling asleep, middle-of-the-night waking, and unrefreshing sleep despite adequate time in bed. These issues were affecting her cognitive function, mood, and overall health.

Initial Challenges: "I'd struggled with sleep for years, trying everything from meditation apps to prescription medications. I could usually fall asleep eventually but would wake around 2–3 a.m. and spend hours tossing and turning. I was functional but never felt truly rested, and it was affecting every aspect of my life, from work performance to personal relationships."

Red Light Protocol: Jennifer began with a medium-sized panel device offering both wavelengths:

Initial protocol:

- 15-minute sessions, 2 hours before bedtime
- Primary focus on chest, abdomen, and face at 12–18 inches
- Red wavelength emphasis (660 nm)
- 4–5 times weekly
- Combined with reduced blue light exposure in evenings

Evolution and Adjustments

1. Extended to 20-minute sessions

2. Added focus on back of neck and head for 5 minutes

3. Incorporated deep breathing exercises during sessions

4. Developed post-session routine: herbal tea, reading with amber glasses, complete darkness

Three-Month Results

- Sleep onset time reduced from average 45–60 minutes to 15–20 minutes

- Nighttime awakenings decreased from 3–4 to 1–2 on average

- Return to sleep time after awakening improved dramatically

- Morning refreshment rating improved from 4/10 to 7/10

- Dream recall increased, suggesting improved REM sleep

- Sleep efficiency (measured by wearable device) increased from 76% to 89%

Key Insights from Jennifer: "The timing was absolutely critical—I experimented with different times and found that 90 minutes to 2 hours before bed was my personal sweet spot. Any closer to bedtime and I felt somewhat energized rather than relaxed. What surprised me most was how the benefits built over time; the first week showed modest improvements, but by week six, my sleep had transformed."

Common Patterns Across Success Stories

While each person's experience was unique, certain patterns emerged across these diverse case studies:

1. The Consistency Factor

Every successful case involved strict adherence to a regular schedule, particularly during the initial 60–90 days. Those who reported the most significant benefits were those who maintained 90%+ consistency with their protocol.

2. The Compounding Timeline

Most participants described a similar pattern of results:

- Weeks 1–2: Subtle, often temporary improvements
- Weeks 3–6: More noticeable and lasting changes
- Months 2–3: Significant improvements that others began noticing

- Months 4–6: Deepening and stabilizing of benefits
- Beyond 6 months: Continued gradual improvement with consistent use

3. The Personalization Progression

Virtually all successful users evolved their protocols through systematic experimentation:

1. Starting with standard recommendations
2. Making single variable changes and tracking results
3. Observing body responses and patterns
4. Developing personalized timing, positioning, and complementary practices
5. Creating seasonal or situational variations as needed

4. The Synergy Effect

The most dramatic results occurred when red light therapy was combined strategically with complementary approaches:

- Proper hydration (mentioned by 80% of successful users)
- Targeted nutritional support
- Appropriate physical activity

- Stress management practices
- Optimized sleep habits

5. The Holistic Expansion

Many users reported benefits extending beyond their initial target concerns:

- Those focusing on skin saw energy improvements
- Those targeting pain experienced mood enhancement
- Those addressing sleep noticed cognitive benefits
- Those focusing on performance found emotional resilience

This suggests that the fundamental cellular mechanisms activated by red light therapy can create cascading benefits across multiple body systems.

Lessons for Your Journey

Based on these case studies, here are key principles to apply to your own red light therapy practice:

1. **Document your baseline thoroughly:** Detailed "before" measurements provide motivation when progress seems slow.

2. **Commit to a minimum of 90-day consistency:** The most significant benefits often emerge after the 60-day mark.

3. **Make singular, methodical adjustments:** Change one variable at a time and track results for at least one week before adjusting again.

4. **Look for complementary practices:** Identify synergistic approaches specific to your primary goals.

5. **Track unexpected benefits:** Some of the most valuable improvements may occur in areas you weren't directly targeting.

6. **Find your personal timing:** Time of day matters significantly, but the optimal window varies by individual and goal.

7. **Embrace the experimental mindset:** Approach your practice with curiosity rather than rigid expectations.

In the next chapter, we'll address common challenges, questions, and troubleshooting techniques to help you overcome any obstacles in your red light therapy journey.

Chapter 9: Troubleshooting and FAQs– Overcoming Common Challenges

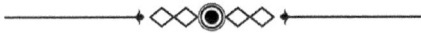

◆◇◇◉◇◇◆

Even with the best devices and protocols, challenges can arise on your red light therapy journey. This chapter addresses the most common obstacles people encounter and provides practical solutions to keep you on track for optimal results.

I've compiled these troubleshooting strategies from thousands of user experiences, clinical observations, and expert interviews. Whether you're just starting out or looking to refine an established practice, these solutions will help you navigate any roadblocks you might face.

Challenge #1: "I'm not seeing results despite consistent use."

This is perhaps the most common concern, especially during the first few weeks. Before assuming the therapy isn't working for you, consider these potential solutions:

Potential Solutions

Insufficient power output

- Verify your device's actual irradiance (mW/cm^2) at your treatment distance.

- Many budget devices deliver far less power than advertised.

- Ensure you're receiving at least 20–30 mW/cm^2 for therapeutic effects.

- Consider decreasing your treatment distance temporarily to increase irradiance.

Inadequate treatment time

- Most common protocols err on the conservative side.

- Try gradually increasing session duration by 25–50%.

- Example: If using 10-minute sessions, try extending to 15 minutes.

- Monitor for any signs of overtreatment (excessive fatigue, irritation).

Suboptimal wavelengths for your specific goal

- Verify your device provides the optimal wavelengths for your target concern:
  - Skin concerns: 630–660 nm (red) is often primary.

o Deep tissue/joints: 810–850 nm (near-infrared) penetrates deeper.

o General wellness: Combination of both wavelengths typically works best.

- If your device offers wavelength options, experiment with different settings.

Inconsistent positioning

- Small variations in distance, angle, or body positioning can significantly affect results.

- Create a consistent setup with measured distances and marked positions.

- Consider using a stand or mounting system rather than hand-holding.

- Maintain the same positioning session-to-session for better tracking.

Unrealistic timeline expectations

- Review the typical timeline for your specific goal (from Chapter 3).

- Some benefits take significantly longer to manifest visibly:

o Skin: Initial glow (days), texture (weeks), wrinkle reduction (months)

o Pain: Temporary relief (days), lasting changes (weeks to months)

- o Hair: Reduced shedding (weeks), visible new growth (months)
- Consider tracking more subtle progress markers

Success Story: James struggled with seeing results for his knee pain despite four weeks of consistent use. After measuring his device's actual output and discovering it was only delivering about 15 mW/cm² at his typical distance, he decreased his treatment distance from 12 inches to 8 inches, effectively doubling the power reaching his knee. Within two weeks of this adjustment, he began experiencing significant pain reduction.

Challenge #2: "I started seeing benefits, but they've plateaued."

Hitting a plateau after initial success is normal but frustrating. Here's how to break through:

Potential Solutions

Protocol cycling

- Your body adapts to consistent stimuli over time
- Try alternating between different protocols:
  - o Vary treatment times (shorter/longer sessions)

- o Change treatment frequency (daily vs. every other day)
- o Alternate wavelengths if your device offers options

- Use a 3:1 approach: three weeks on standard protocol, one week with variations

Position rotation

- Even small changes in angle or position can stimulate different tissues.

- Develop a rotation system for treating the same area from different angles.

- Example for knee treatment: anterior (front), posterior (back), medial (inner), lateral (outer).

- Create a simple diagram to track positioning variations.

Timing adjustments

- Bodily systems respond differently based on time of day.

- If you've been using red light therapy exclusively in the evenings, try mornings.

- Consider splitting into two shorter sessions at different times.

- Align with natural body rhythms (recovery processes peak at different times).

Strategic breaks

- Continuous use can sometimes lead to adaptation.

- Try a 3–5 day complete break, then resume normal protocol.

- Often returns with renewed sensitivity to benefits.

- Consider scheduling regular "rest periods" every 6–8 weeks.

Complementary practice addition

- Add a new synergistic practice to enhance your results:
  - For skin: Exfoliation, hydration focus, specific nutrients.
  - For pain: Contrast therapy, targeted movement, anti-inflammatory nutrition.
  - For energy: Circadian optimization, morning sunlight, stress management.

- Select one complementary practice and implement consistently for 2+ weeks.

Success Story: After three months of excellent results for skin rejuvenation, Elena hit a plateau where improvements seemed to stall. By implementing a rotation system (week 1: standard protocol, week 2: longer sessions at greater distance, week 3: standard protocol, week 4: shorter, more frequent sessions), she broke through the plateau and continued seeing improvements. She also added a gentle exfoliation routine twice weekly, which seemed to enhance light penetration and results.

Challenge #3: "I experience discomfort during or after sessions."

Some discomfort can signal the need for protocol adjustments rather than indicating the therapy isn't right for you.

Potential Solutions

Eye discomfort or sensitivity

- While red/NIR light is generally eye-safe at therapeutic intensities, sensitivity varies.

- Try closing your eyes during treatment (effective for most people).

- Consider specialized eye protection designed for red light therapy.

- Adjust device positioning to reduce direct eye exposure.

- Decrease session duration temporarily, then gradually increase.

Skin irritation or excessive redness

- Increase treatment distance by 25–50%.

- Reduce session duration initially, then gradually build back up.

- Ensure skin is clean but not over-exfoliated before treatment.

- Check for potentially photosensitizing ingredients in skincare products.

- Consider focusing more on near-infrared wavelengths temporarily.

Headaches after treatment

- Often related to dehydration—increase water intake before and after.

- Try shorter sessions with gradual duration increases.

- For transcranial applications, reduce intensity and frequency.

- Consider splitting sessions (morning/evening) rather than one longer session.

- Monitor environment for other triggers (sound, posture during treatment).

Fatigue following sessions

- May indicate mild overtreatment—reduce frequency or duration.

- Consider timing adjustments (morning sessions for energy, evening for sleep).

- Check hydration status and overall health factors.

- Monitor patterns—temporary fatigue followed by energy improvement can be normal.

- Rule out coincidental factors unrelated to treatment.

Success Story: Morgan experienced mild headaches after her initial transcranial sessions for cognitive support. Rather than abandoning the therapy, she reduced session time from 15 to 5 minutes, dramatically increased water intake before and after, and gradually built back up by adding 2 minutes each week. The headaches resolved completely by week three, and she eventually reached 20-minute sessions with no discomfort and significant cognitive benefits.

Challenge #4: "I can't maintain consistency with my protocol."

Consistency challenges are common but solvable with the right strategies.

Potential Solutions

Schedule integration issues

- Anchor treatment to existing daily habits (morning coffee, evening reading, etc.)

- Start with shorter, more manageable sessions (even 5 minutes is beneficial)

- Consider device placement for convenience (bathroom, bedside table, office)

- Prepare a dedicated space where setup time is minimized

- Schedule specific times on calendar with reminders

Motivation fluctuations

- Set clearer short-term goals with visible metrics

- Take baseline photos and measurements for comparison

- Create a visual tracking system (calendar, app, journal)

- Find an accountability partner also using red light therapy
- Join online communities focused on red light therapy for support

Travel and disruptions

- Invest in a travel-friendly device for continuity
- Develop a minimal effective protocol for disrupted periods
- Create specific "travel" or "disruption" protocols (shorter but still effective)
- Plan for double sessions before and after known disruptions
- Focus on highest-priority treatment areas during limited time

Boredom or perceived inconvenience

- Pair sessions with enjoyable activities (audiobooks, podcasts, meditation)
- Create a more pleasant treatment environment (comfortable seating, relaxing space)
- Add variety with different treatment positions or focuses

- Track specific metrics to maintain motivation through visible progress
- Remind yourself of initial goals and documented improvements

Success Story: Jason struggled with maintaining his evening protocol due to unpredictable work hours and family responsibilities. He switched to a morning approach, placing his device in the bathroom to use during his existing morning routine.

Chapter 10: The Sustainable Glow–
Making Red Light a Lifelong Habit

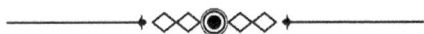

Throughout this book, we've explored the science of red light therapy, practical protocols, and troubleshooting strategies. But perhaps the most important question remains: How do you turn this powerful practice into a sustainable, lifelong habit that continues to serve your health for years to come?

Many wellness practices follow a predictable pattern. We start with enthusiasm, maintain consistency for a few weeks or months, then gradually drift away as life intervenes or initial motivation fades. This pattern is so common that the health and fitness industry actually depends on it—counting on most people to purchase equipment or memberships they'll eventually stop using.

I want something different for you. I want red light therapy to become an enduring practice that delivers cumulative benefits throughout your life, not just another abandoned health gadget gathering dust in a closet.

In this final chapter, we'll explore strategies for long-term sustainability, adapting your practice as you age, staying current with evolving research, and integrating red light therapy into a comprehensive approach to optimal health.

Beyond the 30-Day Kickstart: Creating Your Sustainable Rhythm

The 30-day kickstart plan gave you a structured introduction to red light therapy. Now, let's design a sustainable long-term approach that works with your life rather than demanding your life work around it.

Finding Your Minimum Effective Dose

While more intensive protocols are appropriate when beginning or addressing specific concerns, long-term sustainability often depends on finding your personal minimum effective dose (MED)— the smallest regular investment that maintains your results.

How to Find Your MED

1. After achieving your initial goals, gradually reduce frequency while maintaining session quality:

   o If using daily, try 5 days weekly for 2 weeks

   o If results maintain, try 4 days weekly for 2 weeks

   o Continue until you notice slight regression in benefits

2. When slight regression occurs, return to the previous frequency—this is likely your maintenance MED

3. Similarly, experiment with session duration:

   o Reduce by 25% (e.g., from 20 to 15 minutes)

   o Maintain for 2 weeks and assess results

   o Continue adjusting until finding minimum effective time

4. Document your findings—your personal MED may differ across goals:

   o Skin benefits might maintain with 3x weekly sessions

   o Joint pain might require 4–5x frequency

   o Energy benefits might need briefer but more frequent sessions

Many long-term users find that after initial intensive use, they can maintain most benefits with 3–4 weekly sessions of 10–15 minutes each. This creates a sustainable time investment of 30–60 minutes weekly rather than 15–20 minutes daily.

Integrating Red Light Therapy Into Your Life Rhythms

Rather than viewing red light therapy as something separate you must add to your life, look for natural integration points within your existing routines.

Natural Integration Strategies

Morning routines

- During morning coffee preparation
- While reviewing day or checking emails
- During morning stretching or mobility work
- While listening to news or educational content
- As part of meditation or breathwork practice

Workday integration

- During lunch break relaxation
- While on non-video conference calls

- As a physical/mental reset between tasks
- During afternoon energy dip periods
- As part of standing desk routine

Evening integration

- During evening news or reading time
- While winding down before bed
- During family TV or conversation time
- As part of skincare or self-care routines
- During gentle evening stretching

Effective integrators find existing "windows" where red light therapy enhances rather than competes with established activities. This transforms the practice from "one more thing to do" into "a way to enhance what I'm already doing."

Creating Environmental and Social Support

Your environment significantly impacts habit sustainability. Small adjustments can create powerful cues that support consistent practice.

Environmental design strategies

- **Dedicated space:** Designate a specific area for your device with comfortable seating

- **Visual reminders:** Keep device visible rather than stored away

- **Reduced friction:** Minimize setup time with permanent positioning or easy-access storage

- **Pleasant associations:** Add elements you enjoy to treatment space (plants, artwork, comfortable seating)

- **Session essentials:** Keep items you typically use during sessions (water, reading material, journal) nearby

Social support strategies

- **Shared practice:** Engage family members or housemates in benefits

- **Accountability systems:** Find an accountability partner with similar goals

- **Community connection:** Join online groups focused on red light therapy

- **Progress sharing:** Document and share your journey with supportive friends

- **Expert connection:** Maintain relationship with knowledgeable practitioners

Environmental and social factors often determine habit longevity more than willpower or motivation.

Design your environment to make consistency almost inevitable rather than requiring constant decision-making.

Adapting Your Practice Through Life Stages

As you move through different life stages, your body's needs and responses evolve. A truly sustainable practice adapts accordingly.

Young Adulthood (20s–30s)

During this phase, red light therapy often focuses on:

- Recovery from higher-intensity physical activity
- Prevention rather than correction of skin aging
- Support during high-demand career and family building phases
- Stress management during life transitions
- Optimization of energy and performance

Sustainable approach: Integrate with active lifestyle, emphasizing recovery enhancement, stress management, and preventative benefits. Balance higher-intensity periods with recovery-focused protocols.

Midlife Transitions (40s–50s)

Priorities often shift to:

- Supporting changing hormone patterns
- Addressing emerging joint and muscle concerns
- More focused skin rejuvenation
- Managing energy fluctuations
- Sleep quality enhancement
- Cognitive support for peak professional performance

Sustainable approach: More systematic approach with targeted protocols for emerging concerns. Often benefits from longer sessions with deeper tissue focus (near-infrared). May require more consistent tracking as body signals change.

Active Aging (60s+)

Focus typically evolves toward:

- Maintaining mobility and joint function
- Supporting cellular energy for vitality
- Enhancing circulation and tissue health
- Cognitive maintenance and support
- Skin elasticity and wound healing

- Sleep quality optimization

Sustainable approach: Often benefits from higher-frequency, longer-duration sessions. May require adaptation for changing vision and mobility. Integration with other healthy aging practices becomes increasingly important.

Special Life Transitions

Certain life transitions warrant specific protocol adjustments:

Recovery from major physical events

- Surgery recovery
- Childbirth recovery
- Injury rehabilitation
- Significant weight changes

Hormonal transitions

- Perimenopause/menopause
- Andropause
- Thyroid adaptations
- Stress-related hormonal changes

Each transition represents an opportunity to adapt your practice to provide targeted support when your body needs it most. View these transitions as recalibration points rather than disruptions to your practice.

Staying Current: Navigating Evolving Research and Technology

Red light therapy research and technology continue to evolve rapidly. A sustainable practice includes strategies for staying informed without becoming overwhelmed.

Evaluating New Research

The volume of research on photobiomodulation grows yearly. Here's how to stay reasonably current:

Balanced information sources

- Follow 1–2 research aggregators or knowledgeable practitioners who summarize findings
- Approach manufacturer claims with healthy skepticism
- Look for research patterns rather than single studies
- Consider practical applications rather than just mechanisms
- Distinguish between established benefits and emerging possibilities

Research integration questions: When encountering new research, ask yourself:

1. Has this been replicated in multiple studies?
2. Was it conducted on humans (not just cells or animals)?
3. Does it contradict or enhance current understanding?
4. Does it suggest practical protocol adjustments?
5. Is it relevant to my specific goals?

This framework helps you incorporate valuable new insights without chasing every preliminary finding or theoretical benefit.

Technology Evolution and Upgrades

Red light therapy technology continues advancing. Here's how to approach upgrades wisely:

Signs it's time to consider upgrading

- Your device has limitations directly affecting your primary goals.

- Session time has become prohibitively long due to device limitations.

- New technology offers verified benefits for your specific concerns.

- Your health goals have evolved beyond your current device's capabilities.

- Treatment has become inconvenient enough to affect consistency.

Questions before upgrading

1. Have I optimized my protocol with my current device?

2. Would an accessory or positioning improvement achieve similar benefits?

3. Are the claimed advances supported by independent verification?

4. Will this truly enhance my results or just add complexity?

5. Does the investment align with the importance of my health goals?

Technology improvements can enhance results, but often protocol optimization with existing equipment provides greater benefit than constantly chasing new devices.

Red Light Therapy Within a Comprehensive Health Strategy

While powerful, red light therapy works best as part of an integrated approach to health rather than as an isolated intervention.

Synergistic Daily Practices

Certain daily practices substantially enhance red light therapy's effectiveness:

Hydration practices

- Consistent water intake throughout day
- Mineral balance for cellular hydration
- Additional hydration before and after sessions
- Monitoring hydration status through urine color
- Reduced dehydrating substances (alcohol, excessive caffeine)

Movement integration

- Regular physical activity appropriate for your condition
- Movement breaks throughout sedentary periods
- Mobility work for key joints
- Gentle movement before or during red light sessions
- Recovery-focused movement after intense training

Sleep optimization

- Consistent sleep and wake times
- Appropriate darkness during sleep hours
- Morning light exposure for circadian regulation
- Evening wind-down routines
- Sleep environment optimization

Stress management

- Regular parasympathetic activation
- Breath awareness and regulation
- Mindfulness practices
- Nature exposure
- Social connection and support

These foundational practices create the physiological conditions for optimal red light therapy response while amplifying benefits through complementary mechanisms.

Strategic Nutritional Support

Specific nutritional approaches can enhance particular aspects of red light therapy:

For mitochondrial enhancement

- CoQ10/Ubiquinol

- PQQ (Pyrroloquinoline quinone)
- Magnesium
- B vitamins (especially riboflavin)
- Adequate protein for repair processes

For collagen production and skin benefits

- Vitamin C
- Copper
- Zinc
- Silica
- Amino acid precursors (glycine, proline)

For inflammatory modulation

- Omega-3 fatty acids
- Curcumin/turmeric
- Resveratrol
- Colorful polyphenol-rich foods
- Adequate protein for repair

Rather than taking every supplement mentioned, focus on the categories most relevant to your specific red light therapy goals, prioritizing food-based sources when possible.

The Long View: Cumulative Benefits Over Time

One of red light therapy's most remarkable aspects is how benefits can compound over years of consistent use. Understanding this long-term trajectory helps maintain motivation through inevitable fluctuations.

The Typical Long-Term Timeline

While individual experiences vary, here's a general pattern observed in long-term users:

First 3–6 months

- Most visible and tangible initial benefits emerge.

- Primary targeted concerns show measurable improvement.

- Personal protocol refinement establishes optimal approach.

- Initial excitement may fluctuate as practice becomes routine.

6–12 months

- Deeper, more structural changes become apparent.

- Secondary benefits often emerge beyond initial focus.

- Body adaptation requires periodic protocol adjustment.

- Integration into lifestyle becomes more seamless.

1–3 years

- Cumulative effects create more stable, lasting changes.

- Preventative benefits begin to distinguish from age-matched peers.

- Functional improvements translate to quality of life enhancements.

- Refined intuition about body's needs and responses develops.

3+ years

- Maintenance of benefits that would typically decline with age.

- Increased resilience to stressors and faster recovery from disruptions.

- Personalized expertise about individual response patterns.

- Integration with evolving health needs across life transitions.

Long-term users often report that while initial benefits motivated them to begin, unexpected secondary benefits and general resilience keep them committed years later.

The Cellular Investment Perspective

A helpful framework for long-term motivation is viewing red light therapy as a cellular investment account rather than a quick fix.

Like financial investing, small, consistent contributions compound over time. Each session represents a deposit into your cellular health account, with several parallels to financial investing:

- **Consistency matters more than amount:** Regular small sessions outperform occasional intensive ones.

- **Time in the practice beats timing the practice:** Long-term consistency trumps perfect protocol timing.

- **Diversification provides stability:** Addressing multiple health aspects creates resilience.

- **Compound interest accelerates over time:** Benefits often grow exponentially rather than linearly.

- **Market fluctuations are normal:**
  Response variations are expected and don't
  negate the long-term trend.

- **Panic selling forfeits gains:** Abandoning
  practice during plateaus sacrifices
  accumulated benefits.

- **Professional guidance adds value:**
  Occasional expert consultation enhances
  long-term results.

This perspective helps maintain motivation during
inevitable plateaus by focusing on the long-term
trajectory rather than short-term fluctuations.

Conclusion: Your Light Journey

We've covered considerable ground throughout
this book—from the science behind red light
therapy to practical protocols, troubleshooting
strategies, and now sustainable practice. My goal
has been to provide not just information, but
transformation: a pathway to incorporating this
remarkable technology into your life in a way that
creates lasting benefits.

As you continue your journey with red light therapy, remember these core principles:

1. **Personalization trumps standardization:** Your optimal protocol will ultimately be as unique as your fingerprint, developed through attentive experience rather than rigid rules.

2. **Consistency outweighs perfection:** The best protocol is the one you'll actually follow consistently, even if it's not theoretically optimal.

3. **Integration enhances sustainability:** Rather than treating red light therapy as separate from your life, weave it into existing patterns and priorities.

4. **Curiosity serves better than certainty:** Maintain an experimental mindset, continuously refining your approach based on results rather than preconceptions.

5. **Community accelerates progress:** Connect with others on similar journeys to share insights, maintain motivation, and navigate challenges.

Light has been our constant companion throughout human evolution—signaling our circadian rhythms, providing energy for food production, and guiding our activities. In many ways, therapeutic light applications represent a return to our fundamental relationship with this essential element, harnessing specific wavelengths with intentionality for optimal function.

I invite you to carry forward this practice with patience, consistency, and curiosity. The most profound benefits often emerge not from perfect protocols but from the accumulated wisdom of your own experience—listening to your body, adapting to its changing needs, and maintaining the gentle discipline of showing up for your health day after day, year after year.

May your journey with red light therapy bring lasting illumination to your health and vitality for years to come.

Conclusion

---◆◇◇◉◇◇◆---

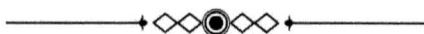

As we reach the end of our journey together, I hope you've gained not only knowledge about red light therapy but also a genuine sense of possibility and empowerment. From understanding the cellular mechanisms of photobiomodulation to creating your personalized protocol, you now possess the tools to harness this remarkable technology for your own well-being.

Throughout this book, we've explored how specific wavelengths of light can influence your cells' energy production, reduce inflammation, enhance collagen synthesis, improve sleep quality, and support numerous other biological processes. We've examined how to select the right device, implement effective protocols, and overcome common challenges. We've seen real people transform their health through consistent practice and thoughtful application.

If there is one central message to take away, it is this: Red light therapy isn't just another fleeting wellness trend or quick fix. It represents a fundamental approach to supporting your body's natural healing and optimization processes. The light energy that has nourished life on this planet for billions of years can now be harnessed with precision to address specific health concerns and enhance overall vitality.

The Ripple Effect of Cellular Health

What makes red light therapy particularly remarkable is its far-reaching impact. By improving cellular function at the mitochondrial level, you are not just addressing isolated symptoms; you are enhancing your body's fundamental capacity for energy production, repair, and regeneration. This creates what I call the "ripple effect" of improved cellular health.

When your cells function optimally, they produce more energy, communicate more effectively, and perform their specialized tasks with greater efficiency. This effect ripples outward, affecting tissues, organs, and eventually whole body systems. This is why many long-term users report benefits that extend well beyond their initial areas of focus—better mood alongside skin improvements, enhanced cognitive clarity alongside pain reduction, and improved digestion alongside better sleep.

In a world where health interventions are often narrowly targeted at specific symptoms, red light therapy offers a refreshingly holistic approach that honors the interconnected nature of human physiology.

Beyond Individual Health: The Broader Implications

The potential impact of red light therapy extends beyond individual health to broader societal benefits. Consider these possibilities:

- **Reduced Medication Dependence:** As more people experience successful pain management through red light therapy, we could see a reduced reliance on pain medications, including opioids, along with their associated side effects and addiction risks.

- **Improved Aging Experience:** By supporting skin health, joint mobility, energy levels, and cognitive function, red light therapy has the potential to transform how we experience aging, allowing for greater vitality and independence in our later years.

- **Sustainable Healthcare:** Home-based red light therapy represents a sustainable health practice with minimal ongoing costs, no consumable products or waste, and the potential to reduce healthcare utilization for manageable conditions.

- **Democratized Health Optimization:** Once limited to elite athletes and expensive clinics, red light therapy is becoming increasingly accessible, enabling more people to experience its benefits regardless of socioeconomic status.

As technology continues to advance and prices decrease, these broader implications may become increasingly significant in the years to come.

The Future of Light Therapy

We're witnessing a renaissance in light-based healing approaches, with red light therapy at the forefront. Research continues to expand into exciting new applications, and technology is evolving to make treatment more efficient, convenient, and personalized.

Emerging areas of interest include:

- Enhanced protocols combining multiple wavelengths for synergistic effects.

- More sophisticated pulse patterns to optimize cellular response.

- Targeted applications for neurological conditions.

- Integration with digital health technologies for personalized dosing and tracking.

- Combination with other treatment modalities for enhanced outcomes.

While we can't predict exactly how the field will evolve, one thing is certain: we're only beginning to understand the full potential of therapeutic light.

Your Role as a Pioneer

By incorporating red light therapy into your health practices, you are joining a growing community of pioneers exploring the intersection of ancient wisdom and cutting-edge science. The knowledge you gain through your personal experience contributes to our collective understanding of this remarkable therapy.

I encourage you to:

- Share your experiences with others who might benefit.

- Stay informed about new research and developments.

- Maintain an experimental mindset, continuing to refine your approach.

- Connect with the broader community of red light therapy users.

- Consider participating in citizen science initiatives or research studies when possible.

Your journey matters not just for your own health but also as part of a larger movement rediscovering the healing potential of light.

A Final Thought: The Simplicity of Light

There is something beautifully elegant about using light for healing. Unlike complex pharmaceuticals or invasive procedures, light therapy works with your body's natural processes in a gentle yet powerful way. It connects us to one of the most fundamental relationships in nature—that between living organisms and light energy.

Whether you are addressing specific health concerns or simply optimizing your well-being, remember that patience and consistency are your greatest allies. The most profound benefits often emerge not from perfect protocols but from the accumulated wisdom of your own experience—listening to your body, adapting to its changing needs, and maintaining the gentle discipline of showing up for your health day after day, year after year.

Thank you for joining me on this exploration of red light therapy. It has been my privilege to guide you through this fascinating field, and I look forward to hearing about your own illuminating journey toward better health.

Bonus: Your Complete Red Light Therapy Toolkit

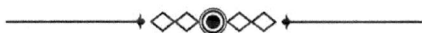

———— ✦◇◇◉◇◇✦ ————

Welcome to the bonus section of *Red Light Therapy: Unlock the Hidden Power of Red Light for Pain Relief, Energy, and Anti-Aging.* These resources represent the practical heart of this book—tools designed to help you implement everything you've learned and achieve meaningful results as quickly as possible.

I have created these bonuses based on the questions, challenges, and needs I have observed from thousands of red light therapy users over the years. They address the most common obstacles people face when beginning their red light journey: Uncertainty about protocols, difficulty tracking progress, confusion about device selection, and trouble maintaining consistency.

Think of these resources as your personal implementation system—transforming knowledge into action and results. Whether you are a detail-oriented planner who wants exact protocols, a visual learner who benefits from clear comparisons, or someone who needs structured tracking to stay motivated, you will find tools specifically designed for your needs.

Inside, you'll discover:

- **The 30-Day Quick-Start Guide:** A day-by-day roadmap that eliminates guesswork and builds momentum through daily wins.

- **The Device Comparison Chart:** Clear specifications and honest assessments to help you find the perfect device for your needs and budget.

- **Treatment Protocol Cheat Sheets:** Precise, condition-specific protocols developed from both research and real-world experience.

- **Progress Tracking Worksheets:** Customizable templates to document your journey and celebrate improvements.

- **Troubleshooting Guide:** Solutions to the most common challenges, helping you overcome obstacles before they derail your progress.

- **Access to the Online Resource Library:** Expanding your toolkit with video demonstrations, expert interviews, and additional resources.

These bonuses aren't afterthoughts; they're the practical bridges between understanding red light therapy and experiencing its benefits in your own life. Many readers tell me they refer to these resources more frequently than the main chapters, especially as they move from learning to implementing.

I encourage you not just to read these resources but to actively use them. Print the worksheets, keep the cheat sheets handy, reference the device guide before purchasing, and follow the 30-day plan step by step. The readers who experience the most dramatic results are invariably those who implement these tools consistently.

30-Day Quick-Start Guide

This 30-Day Quick-Start Guide condenses the essential elements of effective red light therapy into a structured daily program. By following this plan consistently, you will establish the foundation for remarkable results in pain relief, skin health, energy enhancement, recovery, and more.

Week 1: Establishing the Foundation (Days 1–7)

Day 1: Equipment Setup and First Session

- **Morning Task:** Unpack your device, read all manufacturer instructions, and set up your dedicated space.

- **First Session:** 5 minutes at recommended distance on a single area (abdomen or upper back).

- **Evening Reflection:** Note any immediate sensations or effects in your tracking journal.

- **Key Focus:** Familiarization with your device and comfort with the process.

Day 2: Expanding Exposure

- **Morning Task:** Prepare your treatment space with comfortable seating and a timer.

- **Session:** 8 minutes per area on two treatment areas (repeat yesterday's area plus one new area).

- **Evening Reflection:** Compare today's experience to yesterday.

- **Key Focus:** Establishing comfort with longer exposure time.

Day 3: Timing Optimization

- **Morning Task:** Schedule your session at the ideal time for your primary goal.
  - ○ Energy & metabolism: Within 1 hour of waking.
  - ○ Pain relief: Whenever pain typically peaks.
  - ○ Sleep improvement: 1–2 hours before bedtime.

- **Session:** 10 minutes per area on the same two areas as Day 2.

- **Evening Reflection:** How did session timing affect your experience?

- **Key Focus:** Finding your optimal treatment time.

Day 4: Observation Day

- **Morning Task:** No red light session today.

- **Alternative Activity:** Review your notes from the first three days.

- **Evening Reflection:** Notice any lingering effects without treatment.

- **Key Focus:** Developing body awareness and establishing baseline.

Day 5: Target-Specific Application

- **Morning Task:** Identify your primary treatment goal.

- **Session:** 10 minutes on general areas + 10 minutes on primary concern area:
  - Skin: Face and neck
  - Pain: Specific painful area
  - Energy: Abdomen and chest
  - Sleep: Upper back and chest
  - Hair: Scalp

- **Evening Reflection:** Note differences in response between areas.

- **Key Focus:** Precision application for specific concerns.

Day 6: Distance Optimization

- **Morning Task:** Set up measurement markers for consistent positioning.

- **Session:** 10 minutes per area with experimental distances.
  - First area: Slightly closer than previous days.

    o Second area: Slightly farther than previous days.

- **Evening Reflection:** Which distance provided the most comfortable warmth sensation?

- **Key Focus:** Finding your personal sweet spot for treatment distance.

Day 7: First Assessment

- **Morning Task:** Review week one experiences and note initial observations.

- **Session:** 10 minutes per area using your preferred distance.

- **Evening Reflection:** Complete full self-assessment compared to baseline.

- **Key Focus:** Evaluating your first week and planning adjustments.

Week 2: Optimizing Your Approach (Days 8–14)

Day 8–14: Protocol Refinement

- Gradually increase session duration to 15 minutes.

- Experiment with wavelength settings if your device offers options.

- Test morning vs. evening sessions to determine optimal timing.

- Introduce gentle movement during sessions.

- Try post-activity recovery sessions.

- Add mindful breathing during treatment.

- Complete a second progress assessment.

Week 3: Integration and Expansion (Days 15–21)

Day 15–21: Lifestyle Enhancement

- Enhance hydration before and after sessions.

- Boost circulation with light movement before treatment.

- Focus intensively on your primary concern area.

- Combine evening sessions with relaxation techniques.

- Support results with complementary nutrition.

- Practice intuitive application based on body needs.

- Complete a third progress assessment.

Week 4: Fine-Tuning for Maximum Results (Days 22–30)

Day 22–30: Personalization and Mastery

- Design your personalized ongoing protocol.

- Optimize morning sessions for energy and metabolism.

- Time sessions to enhance physical performance.

- Maximize recovery benefits.

- Fine-tune evening sessions for sleep quality.

- Focus on visible improvements in skin or target concerns.

- Complete the final assessment and establish a maintenance plan.

Final Day Assessment Checklist

- Compare current status to baseline measurements.

- Document visible changes with comparison photos.

- Note improvements in energy, pain, sleep, recovery, and other target areas.

- Identify ongoing frequency and duration requirements for maintenance.

- Create your sustainable long-term plan.

Maintenance Recommendations

General Wellness: 3–4 sessions weekly, 10–15 minutes each

Specific Conditions: 4-5 sessions weekly, 15–20 minutes each

Athletic Performance: 3–5 sessions weekly, timed with training schedule

Skin Rejuvenation: 3–4 sessions weekly, with weekly intensive session

Remember, consistency matters more than perfection. A regular, sustainable practice will yield far better results than occasional intense sessions. Use the tracking worksheets to document your journey and refine your approach based on your body's unique responses.

Device Comparison Chart

Specification	What It Means	Target Range	Why It Matters
Wavelength	The specific color of light measured in nanometers (nm)	Red: 630–660 nm Near-infrared: 810–850 nm	Determines depth of penetration and cellular targets
Irradiance	Power density (mW/cm²) at a specific distance	20–100 mW/cm² at treatment distance	The actual "dose" your tissues receive
Total Power	Overall device output in watts	Varies by device size	Affects treatment area and time required
Treatment Area	Size of surface that emits light	Small: <100cm² Medium: 100–500 cm² Large: >500cm²	Determines how much of your body can be treated at once
EMF Levels	Electromagnetic field emissions	<2 milligauss at treatment distance	Lower is better for long-term safety

Device Categories Comparison

Type	Price Range	Pros	Cons	Best For
Handheld Devices	$30–$300	Portable Affordable Good for targeted treatment Easy positioning	Small treatment area Often lower power Longer total treatment time Hand fatigue during use	Beginners Facial applications Travel Spot treatment
Mask/Contoured Devices	$100–$900	Hands-free operation Consistent distance Shaped for specific body parts Comfortable for long sessions	Only treats specific areas Limited versatility Quality varies widely Often lower power	Facial rejuvenation Targeted joint pain Consistent positioning needs Hands-free requirements
Small/Medium Panels	$300–$800	Versatile for different areas Better power output	Still requires multiple sessions for full body	Most home users Multiple treatment areas

RED LIGHT THERAPY

		More efficient treatment time	Less portable	Athletic recovery
		Good value for most users	Requires positioning solutions	Balance of cost/benefit
Large Panels	$800–$2,000	Treats large areas simultaneously	Significant investment	Serious biohackers
		Higher power output	Requires dedicated space	Whole-body benefits
		Most efficient treatment time	Less portable	Multiple users sharing
		Better cooling systems	Higher electricity usage	Maximum efficiency needs
Professional Systems	$2,000–$10,000+	Maximum treatment area	Very high investment	Professional settings
		Highest power output	Requires dedicated space	Multiple daily users
		Advanced controls	Complex operation	Clinical applications
		Optimal efficiency	Designed for clinics	Maximum results priority

Feature Comparison

Feature	Entry-Level	Mid-Range	Premium
Wavelengths	Single wavelength (usually red OR near-infrared)	Dual wavelengths (red AND near-infrared)	Multiple precise wavelengths with independent control
Power Controls	On/off only	Basic timer functions	Programmable sessions, pulsing options, intensity control
LED Quality	Basic consumer-grade LEDs	Medical-grade LEDs	Highest-grade LEDs with optimal lens angles
Cooling System	Passive cooling only	Basic fan cooling	Advanced heat management for extended sessions
Construction	Plastic housing, basic components	Mixed materials, better durability	Medical-grade materials, highest durability
Warranty	0–1 year limited	1–2 year warranty	2+ year comprehensive warranty
Support	Basic documentation only	Email/chat support	Dedicated support team, treatment guidance

Value Assessment Guidelines

- **Budget Priority** ($100–$300): Focus on a quality handheld or small targeted device with verified irradiance of at least 30 mW/cm^2.

- **Balance Priority** ($300–$800): Invest in a medium panel with dual wavelengths and at least 50 mW/cm^2 irradiance.

- **Results Priority** ($800+): Choose a large panel or modular system with independent wavelength control and 75+ mW/cm^2 irradiance.

Remember, the perfect device is one you'll use consistently. Prioritize quality oversize if budget-constrained, as a smaller high-quality device used regularly will outperform a larger low-quality device used occasionally.

Cheat Sheet for Treatment Protocols

General Guidelines for All Applications

- **Hydration:** Drink 8–16oz water before and after sessions for optimal results.

- **Skin Preparation:** Clean skin free of creams, oils, or makeup that could block light.

- **Eyes:** Never stare directly at LEDs; close eyes or use appropriate eyewear if sensitive.

- **Treatment Frequency:** Start with 5–7 sessions weekly for first month, then adjust based on results.

- **Positioning:** Maintain consistent distance between device and treatment area.

- **Timing:** Be consistent with time of day based on your primary goal.

Protocol Framework

Factor	Conservative Approach	Standard Approach	Intensive Approach
Distance	12–18 inches	6–12 inches	4–6 inches
Duration	5–10 minutes per area	10–15 minutes per area	15–20 minutes per area
Frequency	Every other day (3–4×/week)	5–6 times weekly	Twice daily for acute needs
Wavelength	Single wavelength based on target	Combined wavelengths	Layered wavelengths with intensity focus
Best For	Beginners, sensitive individuals	Most applications	Acute conditions, breakthrough needs

Condition-Specific Protocols

Pain and Inflammation Protocols

Acute Joint Pain

- **Distance:** 6–8 inches
- **Duration:** 10–15 minutes per joint
- Frequency: Daily
- **Wavelength Focus:** Near-infrared primary
- **Placement:** Directly over joint plus 2–3 inches surrounding area
- **Special Considerations:** Treat from multiple angles if possible

Chronic Arthritis

- **Distance:** 6–8 inches
- **Duration:** 15–20 minutes per area
- **Frequency:** 5–7 times per week
- **Wavelength Focus:** Balanced wavelengths
- **Placement:** Joint plus surrounding tissues
- **Special Considerations:** Consistent long-term use is critical

Muscle Soreness

- **Distance:** 8–12 inches
- **Duration:** 10–15 minutes per muscle
- **Frequency:** After activity
- **Wavelength Focus:** Near-infrared primary
- **Placement:** Entire muscle belly
- **Special Considerations:** Best when combined with gentle movement

Back Pain

- **Distance:** 6–10 inches
- **Duration:** 15–20 minutes
- Frequency: Daily
- **Wavelength Focus:** Near-infrared primary
- **Placement:** Pain site plus 3–4 inches around
- **Special Considerations:** Multiple angles essential for deep tissue

Nerve Pain

- **Distance:** 6–8 inches
- **Duration:** 15 minutes per area
- **Frequency:** 5–7 times per week

- **Wavelength Focus:** Near-infrared primary
- **Placement:** Follow nerve pathway
- **Special Considerations:** May require 4–6 weeks for significant results

Skin Health Protocols

Anti-Aging

- **Distance:** 6–12 inches
- **Duration:** 10–15 minutes per area
- **Frequency:** 5 times per week
- Wavelength Focus: Red primary
- **Placement:** Face, neck, décolletage
- **Special Considerations:** Remove makeup, apply serums after

Acne

- **Distance:** 6–8 inches
- **Duration:** 10 minutes per area
- Frequency: Daily
- Wavelength Focus: Red primary
- **Placement:** Affected areas

- **Special Considerations:** Clean skin thoroughly before treatment

Wound Healing

- **Distance:** 6–8 inches
- **Duration:** 10 minutes per wound
- **Frequency:** Twice daily
- **Wavelength Focus:** Balanced wavelengths
- **Placement:** Wound plus 1-inch margin
- **Special Considerations:** Do not shine directly on open wounds

Psoriasis/Eczema

- **Distance:** 8–12 inches
- **Duration:** 10–15 minutes per area
- Frequency: Daily
- Wavelength Focus: Red primary
- **Placement:** Affected areas
- **Special Considerations:** Start with reduced time to assess sensitivity

Scars

- **Distance:** 6–8 inches
- **Duration:** 15–20 minutes per area

- Frequency: Daily
- **Wavelength Focus:** Balanced wavelengths
- **Placement:** Directly on scar tissue
- **Special Considerations:** Combine with gentle massage after treatment

Performance and Recovery Protocols

Pre-Workout

- **Distance:** 6–12 inches
- **Duration:** 5–10 minutes per area
- **Frequency:** Before activity
- Wavelength Focus: Red primary
- **Placement:** Target muscle groups
- **Special Considerations:** Use 10–30 minutes before activity

Post-Workout

- **Distance:** 6–12 inches
- **Duration:** 10–15 minutes per area
- **Frequency:** After activity
- **Wavelength Focus:** Near-infrared primary
- **Placement:** Worked muscles

- **Special Considerations:** Use within 1 hour post-exercise

Injury Recovery

- **Distance:** 6–8 inches
- **Duration:** 15–20 minutes per area
- **Frequency:** Twice daily
- **Wavelength Focus:** Balanced wavelengths
- **Placement:** Injury site plus surrounding area
- **Special Considerations:** Consistent application critical

Recovery Day

- **Distance:** 8–12 inches
- **Duration:** 15–20 minutes per area
- **Frequency:** On rest days.
- **Wavelength Focus:** Near-infrared primary
- **Placement:** Large muscle groups
- **Special Considerations:** Full-body session ideal if possible

General Wellness Protocols

Energy Enhancement

- **Distance:** 12–18 inches
- **Duration:** 10–15 minutes
- Frequency: Morning
- **Wavelength Focus:** Balanced wavelengths
- **Placement:** Torso (abdomen/chest)
- **Special Considerations:** Within 1 hour of waking for best results

Sleep Improvement

- **Distance:** 12–18 inches
- **Duration:** 10–15 minutes
- Frequency: Evening
- Wavelength Focus: Red primary
- **Placement:** Upper body, face
- **Special Considerations:** 1–2 hours before bedtime

Mood Support

- **Distance:** 8–12 inches
- **Duration:** 10–15 minutes

- Frequency: Morning
- **Wavelength Focus:** Near-infrared primary
- **Placement:** Head, chest, abdomen
- **Special Considerations:** Combine with deep breathing

Immune Support

- **Distance:** 8–12 inches
- **Duration:** 15 minutes
- Frequency: Daily
- **Wavelength Focus:** Balanced wavelengths
- **Placement:** Chest, throat, abdomen
- **Special Considerations:** Consistency especially important

Brain Function

- **Distance:** 4–8 inches
- **Duration:** 10–15 minutes
- Frequency: Morning
- **Wavelength Focus:** Near-infrared only
- **Placement:** Forehead, temples
- **Special Considerations:** Keep eyes closed, combine with cognitive activity

Tracking and Progress Worksheets

Initial Assessment Worksheet

Personal Information

Name:

Start Date:

Primary Goals:

Device Type & Specifications:

Baseline Measurements

Rate each area from 1–10 (1 = poor, 10 = excellent)

Physical Well-being

- Overall Energy Level: _____
- Morning Energy: _____
- Afternoon Energy: _____
- Evening Energy: _____

- Recovery from Activity: _____
- Sleep Quality: _____
- Time to Fall Asleep: _____ minutes
- Night Awakenings: _____ per night
- Morning Refreshment: _____

Pain Assessment

- Location #1: _____ Pain Level: _____
- Location #2: _____ Pain Level: _____
- Location #3: _____ Pain Level: _____
- Overall Discomfort: _____
- Pain Medication Usage: _____ times per week

Skin Health

- Overall Appearance: _____
- Texture/Smoothness: _____
- Tone/Evenness: _____
- Fine Lines/Wrinkles: _____
- Redness/Inflammation: _____
- Breakouts/Blemishes: _____

- Elasticity/Firmness: _____

Performance Metrics

- Workout Capacity: _____
- Recovery Time: _____ hours
- Endurance Level: _____
- Strength Level: _____
- Flexibility: _____
- Mental Focus: _____
- Cognitive Sharpness: _____

Photo Documentation

Take well-lit photos of target areas from consistent angles:

- Face: Front and both profiles
- Problem skin areas: Direct and angled shots
- Pain/inflammation sites: With measurement reference
- Hair concerns: Top-down and side views
- Body composition: Front, side, and back (if relevant)

Date photos taken: _____

Photo storage location: _____

Daily Session Tracker

Date	Time	Duration	Areas Treated	Distance	Wavelength Setting	Before Session Notes	After Session Notes

Weekly Progress Review

Week: _____

(Dates: _____ to _____)

Session Consistency

- Planned Sessions: _____
- Completed Sessions: _____
- Consistency Rate: _____%

Protocol Adjustments

- Changes made this week:

  _____

- Reason for changes:

  _____

- Effect of changes:

  _____

Physical Changes Observed

- Energy Improvements:

  _____

- Pain Changes:

  _____

- Skin Changes:

  _____

- Performance Changes:

  _____

- Sleep Changes:

  _____

- Other Observations:

  _____

Mental/Emotional Changes

- Mood Shifts:

  _____

- Stress Levels:

  _____

- Mental Clarity:

  _____

- Other Observations:

  _____

Next Week's Plan

- Frequency Adjustments:

  _____

- Duration Adjustments:

  _____

- Focus Areas:

  _____

- Other Strategy Changes:

  _____

30-Day Assessment Summary

Overall Consistency

- Total Planned Sessions: _____
- Total Completed Sessions: _____
- Overall Adherence Rate: _____%

Results By Category

Rate improvement in each area (0 = none, 5 = significant)

Energy and Vitality

- Morning Energy: ___/5
- Afternoon Energy: ___/5
- Evening Energy: ___/5
- Overall Vitality: ___/5
- Specific Changes Noted:

Pain and Inflammation

- Location #1: _____
  Improvement: ___/5
- Location #2: _____
  Improvement: ___/5

- Location #3: _____
  Improvement: ___/5
- Overall Pain Reduction: ___/5
- Medication Changes:

Skin Health
- Overall Appearance: ___/5
- Texture/Smoothness: ___/5
- Tone/Evenness: ___/5
- Fine Lines/Wrinkles: ___/5
- Specific Improvements:

Sleep Quality
- Time to Fall Asleep: ___/5
- Sleep Continuity: ___/5
- Morning Refreshment: ___/5
- Overall Sleep Quality: ___/5
- Specific Changes:

Performance and Recovery
- Workout Capacity: ___/5
- Recovery Speed: ___/5

- Overall Performance: ___/5
- Specific Improvements:

_____

Unexpected Benefits

-
-
-

Comparison Photos

- Date of comparison photos:

  _____

- Notable visible changes:

  _____

- Areas needing more focus:

  _____

Protocol Effectiveness

- Most effective aspect of protocol:

  _____

- Least effective aspect of protocol:

  _____

- Key learnings:

_____

Next Steps

- Maintenance protocol frequency:

_____

- Maintenance session duration:

_____

- Focus areas for continued improvement:

_____

- Additional modalities to incorporate:

_____

Common Mistakes and Troubleshooting Guide

Device Selection Mistakes

Common Mistake	Warning Signs	Solution
Underpowered Device	No warming sensation No results after 4+ weeks Requires extremely long sessions	Verify actual irradiance (mW/cm^2) Decrease treatment distance Consider upgrading to higher power device
Wrong Wavelength	Results in some areas but not target concern Surface benefits only	For deep tissue concerns, ensure device has near-infrared (810–850 nm) For skin concerns, ensure red wavelengths (630–660 nm)
Too Small Treatment Area	Treatment sessions take excessively long Inconsistent results across body	For whole-body benefits, invest in larger panel Create systematic rotation schedule for smaller devices
Poor Quality LEDs	Inconsistent results Early device failure Flickering or dimming during use	Research manufacturer reputation Check LED specifications and origin Invest in better quality device for long-term use

Protocol Implementation Errors

Common Mistake	Warning Signs	Solution
Inconsistent Usage	Minimal or fluctuating results Difficulty tracking progress	Schedule sessions at same time daily Set calendar reminders Link to existing habits (morning coffee, evening routine)
Incorrect Distance	No gentle warming sensation Excessive heat or discomfort Minimal results despite consistent use	Follow manufacturer distance recommendations Create physical markers for consistent positioning Experiment with 25% closer/farther and track results
Insufficient Duration	Minimal results despite consistency Benefits fade quickly	Gradually increase session time by 25–50% Ensure minimum 10–15 minutes per treatment area
Overtreatment	Diminishing returns Fatigue after sessions Skin irritation or sensitivity	Reduce frequency or duration Increase treatment distance Implement 1–2 rest days weekly
Poor Timing	Energy disruption (too stimulated at night or too relaxed when needing energy) Minimal results for specific goals	For energy: morning sessions For sleep: evening sessions (1–2 hours before bed) For pain: time around peak discomfort periods

Treatment Area Mistakes

Common Mistake	Warning Signs	Solution
Treating Through Clothing	Minimal results despite consistency	Always treat bare skin Remove clothing from treatment area
Treating Through Products	Inconsistent or minimal results	Thoroughly cleanse skin before treatment Apply products after treatment
Insufficient Coverage	Incomplete or spotty results	Ensure entire target area receives light Treat 2–3 inches beyond visible problem area Use systematic overlapping approach
Single-Angle Treatment	Deep tissue issues respond poorly Inconsistent results	Treat from multiple angles Rotate position during longer sessions
Ignoring Secondary Areas	Limited systemic benefits	Include torso treatment for whole-body effects Rotate through major body systems

Device Troubleshooting

Issue	Possible Causes	Solutions
Device won't power on	Power connection issue Internal component failure	Check all connections Try different outlet Contact manufacturer
Flickering lights	Loose connection Power supply issue LED failure	Check connections Try different power source Contact manufacturer if persistent
Diminished brightness	Normal LED lifespan degradation Power supply issue	Verify with light meter if possible Clean device surface Contact manufacturer if significant
Unusual noise	Fan obstruction Internal component issue	Ensure ventilation openings clear Contact manufacturer if persistent
Overheating	Blocked ventilation Extended usage beyond rating Internal component issue	Ensure adequate airflow Follow recommended session limits Allow cooling between sessions

Troubleshooting Common Issues

Problem: "I've been consistent but see no results."

Possible Causes

1. Insufficient device power
2. Incorrect wavelength for target concern
3. Treating through clothing or products
4. Insufficient session duration
5. Unrealistic timeline expectations

Solutions

- Verify device specifications (at least 30 mW/cm² at your treatment distance)

- Ensure proper wavelength for your condition (NIR for deep tissue, Red for surface)

- Treat bare skin directly

- Increase session duration by 25–50%

- Review typical timeline for your specific concern (some benefits take 8–12 weeks)

Problem: "I experienced initial benefits that have plateaued."

Possible Causes

1. Body adaptation
2. Protocol stagnation
3. Underlying factors not addressed
4. Natural ceiling of benefits reached

Solutions

- Implement protocol cycling (vary parameters every 3–4 weeks)
- Try "pulse protocol" with intentional 3–5 day breaks every few weeks
- Examine complementary factors (hydration, nutrition, movement, stress)
- Adjust expectations and focus on maintenance

Problem: "I experience discomfort during or after sessions."

Possible Causes

1. Treatment distance too close
2. Session duration too long
3. Sensitivity to treatment
4. Device issues or EMF sensitivity

5. Dehydration

Solutions

- Increase treatment distance by 25–50%

- Reduce session duration until comfortable, then gradually rebuild

- Check for photosensitizing medications or conditions

- Ensure adequate hydration before and after treatment

- Verify device is functioning properly

Problem: "Benefits disappear quickly after sessions."

Possible Causes

1. Insufficient treatment frequency
2. Underlying factors overwhelming benefits
3. Incorrect wavelength for concern
4. Need for more comprehensive approach

Solutions

- Increase session frequency (daily may be necessary for some conditions)

- Address lifestyle factors undermining benefits

- Verify wavelength appropriateness for target concern
- Consider complementary approaches alongside red light therapy

Problem: "I get different results each time."

Possible Causes

1. Inconsistent positioning or distance
2. Variable session timing
3. Fluctuating hydration or physiological state
4. Environmental factors

Solutions

- Create positioning aids for consistent distance
- Standardize time of day for treatments
- Maintain consistent hydration and pre-session routine
- Control environmental factors (temperature, ambient light)

Device Troubleshooting

Issue	Possible Causes	Solutions
Device won't power on	Power connection issue Internal component failure	Check all connections Try different outlet Contact manufacturer
Flickering lights	Loose connection Power supply issue LED failure	Check connections Try different power source Contact manufacturer if persistent
Diminished brightness	Normal LED lifespan degradation Power supply issue	Verify with light meter if possible Clean device surface Contact manufacturer if significant
Unusual noise	Fan obstruction Internal component issue	Ensure ventilation openings clear Contact manufacturer if persistent
Overheating	Blocked ventilation Extended usage beyond rating Internal component issue	Ensure adequate airflow Follow recommended session limits Allow cooling between sessions

Remember, most issues can be resolved with proper device selection, consistent application, and attention to details like treatment distance, duration, and frequency. When in doubt, return to the fundamentals: quality device, proper distance, adequate duration, and consistent frequency.

References

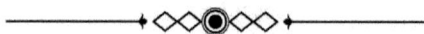

Avci, P., Gupta, A., Sadasivam, M., Vecchio, D., Pam, Z., Pam, N., & Hamblin, M. R. (2013). Low-level laser (light) therapy (LLLT) in skin: Stimulating, healing, restoring. *Seminars in Cutaneous Medicine and Surgery, 32*(1), 41–52.

Chung, H., Dai, T., Sharma, S. K., Huang, Y. Y., Carroll, J. D., & Hamblin, M. R. (2012). The nuts and bolts of low-level laser (light) therapy. *Annals of Biomedical Engineering*, 40(2), 516–533.

de Almeida, P., Lopes-Martins, R. Á., De Marchi, T., Tomazoni, S. S., Albertini, R., Corrêa, J. C., Rossi, R. P., Machado, G. P., da Silva, D. P., Bjordal, J. M., & Leal Junior, E. C. (2012). Red (660 nm) and infrared (830 nm) low-level laser therapy in skeletal muscle fatigue in humans: What is better? *Lasers in Medical Science, 27*(2), 453–458.

Ferraresi, C., Hamblin, M. R., & Parizotto, N. A. (2012). Low-level laser (light) therapy

(LLLT) on muscle tissue: Performance, fatigue and repair benefited by the power of light. *Photonics & Lasers in Medicine, 1*(4), 267–286.

Hamblin, M. R. (2016). Photobiomodulation or low-level laser therapy. *Journal of Biophotonics, 9*(11–12), 1122–1124.

Hamblin, M. R. (2017). Mechanisms and applications of the anti-inflammatory effects of photobiomodulation. *AIMS Biophysics, 4*(3), 337–361.

Heiskanen, V., & Hamblin, M. R. (2018). Photobiomodulation: Lasers vs. light emitting diodes? *Photochemical & Photobiological Sciences, 17*(8), 1003–1017.

Leal-Junior, E. C., Vanin, A. A., Miranda, E. F., de Carvalho, P. T., Dal Corso, S., & Bjordal, J. M. (2015). Effect of phototherapy (low-level laser therapy and light-emitting diode therapy) on exercise performance and markers of exercise recovery: A systematic review with meta-analysis. *Lasers in Medical Science, 30*(2), 925–939.

Salehpour, F., Mahmoudi, J., Kamari, F., Sadigh-Eteghad, S., Rasta, S. H., & Hamblin, M. R. (2018). Brain photobiomodulation therapy:

A narrative review. *Molecular Neurobiology,* *55*(8), 6601-6636.

Sommer, A. P., Pinheiro, A. L., Mester, A. R., Franke, R. P., & Whelan, H. T. (2001). Biostimulatory windows in low-intensity laser activation: Lasers, scanners, and NASA's light-emitting diode array system. *Journal of Clinical Laser Medicine & Surgery,* *19*(1), 29–33.

Vladimirov, Y. A., Osipov, A. N., & Klebanov, G. I. (2004). Photobiological principles of therapeutic applications of laser radiation. *Biochemistry (Moscow), 69*(1), 81–90.

Wang, X., Tian, F., Soni, S. S., Gonzalez-Lima, F., & Liu, H. (2016). Interplay between up-regulation of cytochrome-c-oxidase and hemoglobin oxygenation induced by near-infrared laser. *Scientific Reports*, 6, 30540.

Whelan, H. T., Smits, R. L., Buchman, E. V., Whelan, N. T., Turner, S. G., Margolis, D. A., Cevenini, V., Stinson, H., Ignatius, R., Martin, T., Cwiklinski, J., Philippi, A. F., Graf, W. R., Hodgson, B., Gould, L., Kane, M., Chen, G., & Caviness, J. (2001). Effect of NASA light-emitting diode irradiation on wound healing. *Journal of Clinical Laser Medicine & Surgery, 19*(6), 305–314.

Zein, R., Selting, W., & Hamblin, M. R. (2018). Review of light parameters and photobiomodulation efficacy: Dive into complexity. *Journal of Biomedical Optics, 23*(12), 1–17.

Book Description

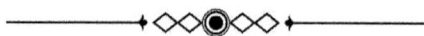

Red Light Therapy: Unlock the Hidden Power of Red Light for Pain Relief, Energy, and Anti-Aging

The practical, no-fluff guide to harnessing the healing power of light

Are you tired of wellness trends that promise miracles but deliver disappointment? Red light therapy is different—a science-backed approach that's transforming how we think about healing, aging, and energy.

In this straightforward, action-focused guide, you'll discover:

- **The Science Made Simple:** Understand exactly how specific wavelengths of light affect your cells without needing a biology degree

- **A Complete 30-Day Action Plan:** Follow a day-by-day program designed to deliver noticeable results in your first month

- **Specific Protocols for Every Need:** Whether you're fighting chronic pain, seeking better skin, boosting energy, improving sleep, or enhancing athletic performance

- **The Exact How-To:** Learn precise timing, positioning, and frequency for maximum benefits

- **Real Results from Real People:** Authentic case studies showing transformations in pain, skin health, energy levels, and more

- **Advanced Strategies:** Break through plateaus with cutting-edge techniques used by health optimization experts

This isn't just another theory book—it's a practical roadmap to using red light therapy effectively. With clear explanations, visual guides, and step-by-step instructions, you'll learn how to select the right device, implement proven protocols, and track your results for meaningful improvements.

Whether you're a biohacker seeking peak performance, someone fighting chronic pain or skin issues, or simply curious about this revolutionary approach to health, this book provides everything you need to start seeing benefits within days, not months.

No hype. No fluff. Just practical guidance for unlocking the remarkable healing potential of red light therapy.

FREE BONUS FROM PEAKSTATE PROTOCOLS

Greetings!

First, thank you for reading our books.

As a welcome gift we offer the Peakstate Protocols eBook Bundle for free. Plus, you can be the first to receive new books and exclusives! Remember it's 100% free to join.

Simply click the link below to join.

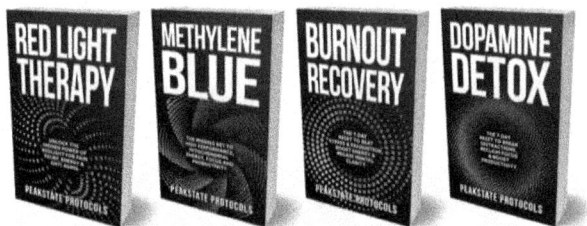

https://www.subscribepage.com/peakstate

Keep up to date with us on:

https://peakstateprotocols.com/

OTHER BOOKS BY PEAKSTATE PROTOCOLS

- Dopamine Detox: The 7-Day Reset to Break Distractions, Reclaim Focus & Boost Productivity

- Red Light Therapy: Unlock the Hidden Power of Redlight for Pain Relief, Energy & Anti-Aging

- Methylene Blue: The Missing Key to High Performance, Mitochondrial Energy, Focus and Productivity

- Burnout Recovery: The 7-Day Reset to Beat Stress & Exhaustion, Boost Energy & Regain Mental Clarity